Praise for *The Anatomy of Medical Errors*

"With unimaginable serenity, Crisp takes us on her Shakespearean journey with superb skill, startling courage, and searing introspection. Her nightmare reveals a frightening level of dysfunction in our increasingly impersonal medical system. In the words of Othello's Desdemona: "These are portents; but yet I hope, I hope, They do not point on me." Those of us in medicine must not ignore either this tragedy, or the heroine who survived it."

–Byers W. Shaw Jr., MD
Professor, Department of Surgery
University of Nebraska Medical Center

"With medical mistakes now our third leading cause of death, I think it's wise for people to become somewhat less afraid of disease and a lot more afraid of treatments."

–Allen Frances, MD
Chair, DSM IV Task Force
Professor Emeritus & Former Chair
Duke University School of Medicine
Department of Psychiatry and Behavioral Sciences
Author, *Saving Normal*

"What a masterpiece! Far beyond a litany of errors, this story could only be written by a nurse who was profoundly betrayed by our health "care" system and by her "care" givers. By courageously sharing her personal story, Donna Helen Crisp gently leads all of us back to our shared humanity. Follow her and you will never be able to see medicine or nursing through the same lens again. Her wisdom, observations, and insight are unparalleled and illuminate the path to healing for both patients and nurses."

–Kathleen Bartholomew, MN, RN
Author, Speaker, and Educator

ANATOMY OF
MEDICAL
ERRORS

THE PATIENT IN ROOM 2

A nurse's story of surviving preventable medical
errors and discovering the truth

DONNA HELEN CRISP, JD, MSN, RN, PMHCNS-BC

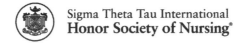

Sigma Theta Tau International
Honor Society of Nursing®

Copyright © 2017 by Donna Helen Crisp

The Honor Society of Nursing, Sigma Theta Tau International (STTI) is a nonprofit organization founded in 1922 whose mission is advancing world health and celebrating nursing excellence in scholarship, leadership, and service. Members include practicing nurses, instructors, researchers, policymakers, entrepreneurs, and others. STTI has more than 500 chapters located at more than 700 institutions of higher education throughout Armenia, Australia, Botswana, Brazil, Canada, Colombia, England, Ghana, Hong Kong, Japan, Kenya, Lebanon, Malawi, Mexico, the Netherlands, Pakistan, Portugal, Singapore, South Africa, South Korea, Swaziland, Sweden, Taiwan, Tanzania, Thailand, the United Kingdom, and the United States of America. More information about STTI can be found online at www.nursingsociety.org.

Sigma Theta Tau International
550 West North Street
Indianapolis, IN, USA 46202

To order additional books, buy in bulk, or order for corporate use, contact Nursing Knowledge International at 888.NKI.4YOU (888.654.4968/US and Canada) or +1.317.634.8171 (outside US and Canada).

To request a review copy for course adoption, email solutions@nursingknowledge.org or call 888.NKI.4YOU (888.654.4968/US and Canada) or +1.317.634.8171 (outside US and Canada).

To request author information, or for speaker or other media requests, contact Marketing, Honor Society of Nursing, Sigma Theta Tau International at 888.634.7575 (US and Canada) or +1.317.634.8171 (outside US and Canada).

ISBN: 9781940446844
EPUB ISBN: 9781940446851
PDF ISBN: 9781940446868
MOBI ISBN: 9781940446875

Library of Congress Cataloging-in-Publication data

Names: Crisp, Donna Helen, 1947- author. I Sigma Theta Tau International, issuing body.
Title: Anatomy of medical errors : the patient in room 2 : a nurse's story of surviving preventable medical errors and discovering the truth / Donna Helen Crisp.
Description: Indianapolis, IN : Sigma Theta Tau International, [2017] I Includes bibliographical references. I Description based on print version record and CIP data provided by publisher; resource not viewed.
Identifiers: LCCN 2016021297 (print) I LCCN 2016020941 (ebook) I ISBN 9781940446851 (Epub) I ISBN 9781940446868 (Pdf) I ISBN 9781940446875 (Mobi) I ISBN 9781940446844 (print : alk. paper) I ISBN 9781940446851 (EPUB) I ISBN 9781940446868 (PDF) I ISBN 9781940446875 (MOBI)
Subjects: I MESH: Medical Errors I Hysterectomy I Intraoperative Complications I Malpractice I Patient Harm I Nurses I Personal Narratives
Classification: LCC R729.8 (print) I LCC R729.8 (ebook) I NLM WP 468 I DDC 610.28/9--dc23
LC record available at https://lccn.loc.gov/2016021297

First Printing, 2016

PUBLISHER: Dustin Sullivan
ACQUISITIONS EDITOR: Emily Hatch
EDITORIAL COORDINATOR: Paula Jeffers
COVER DESIGNER: Rebecca Batchelor
BOOK DESIGN & LAYOUT: Rebecca Batchelor

DEVELOPMENT AND PROJECT EDITOR: Carla Hall
COPY EDITOR: Meaghan O'Keeffe
PROOFREADERS: Jane Palmer, Erin Geile, Nancy Sixsmith

DEDICATION

To my mother and father,
who taught me to fight for justice.

To my family and Shakespeare,
who taught me to love words.

ACKNOWLEDGMENT

Without my conjuring up his brilliance with language and plot, William Shakespeare became part of my writing journey from the beginning of this project. With no thought or intention to use anyone's quotations, I somehow felt compelled to consult Shakespeare, beginning in the early days, when I first began to write down the details of what happened to me.

Throughout the years of writing this book, I did not tell Shakespeare to stay or to go away. I just observed his presence along every twist and turn of my writing. Only in the final stages of completing my manuscript did I begin to think of my story as a true tragedy. Then, it made sense that Shakespeare, a master of tragedy, had helped me tell my story. I am grateful for his inspiration and honored for his assistance.

ABOUT THE AUTHOR

Donna Helen Crisp, JD, MSN, RN, PMHCNS-BC, grew up in Raleigh, North Carolina, the oldest of five daughters. Her father was an attorney, pianist, and poet. Her mother was a psychologist, actress, and writer. After earning a bachelor of arts in English from North Carolina State University, Crisp worked as a social worker until she attended North Carolina Central University School of Law to earn her juris doctor. She then worked as a legal writer, singer-songwriter, French teacher, and restaurant manager before attending the University of North Carolina (UNC) School of Nursing in Chapel Hill, where she earned both her bachelor of science in nursing and her master of science in mental health nursing.

Crisp became board certified in adult psychiatry in 1997. Since then, she has worked with clients challenged with mental illness, dementia, alcohol and substance abuse, and other chronic conditions in various nursing settings, including hospitals, long-term care facilities, clinics, homes, and private practice. Her nursing care has focused on the suffering of her patients and their quality of life.

Of all her professional roles in nursing, Crisp has derived the greatest satisfaction from working with patients and with students. After teaching in the community college system, she became an assistant professor at UNC's School of Nursing in Chapel Hill, where she taught in the undergraduate and graduate programs. In 2008, students honored her as a "most influential leader" for her outstanding guidance, inspiration, and nursing excellence. Her areas of expertise include mental illness, suffering, and ethical decision-making. She has presented on these topics and more at numerous conferences.

As a nurse, Crisp has served her community in various roles, including as chair of the Dementia Community Path Team for western North Carolina, as a member of two hospital ethics committees, and as a member-consultant of the North Carolina Medical Society's Ethical and Judicial Affairs Committee. She has researched and published on various topics, including advance directives and chronic illness. Her abiding passion continues to focus on recognition and amelioration of suffering wherever it exists.

Retired from UNC, Crisp lives in Asheville, North Carolina, with her two Welsh Corgis, Nellie and Ava, and one rescue cat, Clooney. Currently, she is working part time as a nurse and planning her next book.

TABLE OF CONTENTS

TABLE OF CONTENTS

FOREWORD

*"If you have tears
prepare to shed them now"*
–*Julius Caesar*, Act 3. Scene 2

What a story and what a magnificent writer. Donna Helen Crisp tells a story that is unbelievable and, at the same time, captivating and heartbreaking. She is inspired not only by Shakespeare as her muse—and the timeless fates of humanity—but also by her dramatic and inconceivable experiences as a patient.

What this book uncovers needs to be made known to the world of patients, healthcare practitioners, healthcare systems, and the larger public. This work is so revealing and so honest in its exposé that all of us in healthcare must admit and surrender to the painful truth of our current callous, corporate model of human health and treatment—whereby the body becomes reduced to the moral status of an object and is no longer a human being.

The author, a vibrant, healthy woman, is innocent and trusting. When she yields to the dominant paradigm, she learns firsthand the reality of medical errors and, perhaps even more importantly, the accompanying disregard of her basic humanity—the disrespect, dehumanization, and dismissive concerns of her, the human on the other side of healthcare.

Crisp's story, as powerful and painful as it is to read, mirrors what could be anyone's story, anyone's reality, anyone's tragedy. Her story shines a bright light to expose the dominant corporate medical establishment. She highlights the unyielding status quo and the unwillingness of the dominant system to see itself and remedy its inhumane approach to medicine and healthcare. No care, instead of healthcare, occurs in those intimate moments of treatment (at all costs) and the larger protective culture.

Anatomy of Medical Errors dissects the details as well as the landscape of our broken health/sick care model, a system that places treatment and cure at all costs above any concerns for what is at stake— except, perhaps, saving the egos of practitioners and hospitals that are protected by the underbelly of denial against the true story behind the scenes.

Reading this book is scary, and being a silent, vicarious witness hurts as she takes us into the inferno of her personal journey. Planned and structured as an outpatient procedure, her journey becomes an unending nightmare. It churns my heart, as it will the heart of any one who reads this work.

I am grateful to Donna Helen Crisp for her courage, truth-seeking, and willingness to speak out, as well as for her writing talents and gifts she offers as timeless teachings—if we can only listen and learn from her lessons.

–Jean Watson, PhD, RN, AHN-BC, FAAN,
Living Legend AAN
Founder/Director, Watson Caring Science Institute
Distinguished Professor and Dean Emerita
University of Colorado Denver
www.watsoncaringscience.org

PROLOGUE

*"My tongue will tell the anger of my heart
or else my heart, concealing it, will break"*
–The Taming of the Shrew, Act 4, Scene 3

No one ever acknowledged or apologized for the medical errors that changed my life. I came out of a long coma and off the ventilator in a surgical intensive care unit (SICU) at a large teaching hospital with no idea where I was, much less what had happened to me. Although temporarily psychotic and hallucinating, I was somehow able to form one important rational thought: I had to survive and get out of the hospital so I could discover what almost killed me. Then, I had to share my story so others might learn from my tragedy. I did not realize it would take years to learn how I ended up unconscious and dying in a hospital for weeks instead of coming home the day after admission as planned.

Along the way, I learned the truth about medical errors inside hospitals. The Institute of Medicine's (IOM) 1999 report, *To Err Is Human*, generated a national conversation when it reported that 98,000 people die each year because of medical errors in hospitals (Kohn, Corrigan, & Donaldson, 2000). The initial reaction from the medical community was disbelief, dispute, and argument over the numbers. However, hospitals eventually became less critical of this terrifying statistic, though they did little to adequately address the problem that has continued to grow worse.

A 2012 report (Andel, Davidow, Hollander, & Moreno) published in the *Journal of Health Care Finance* suggested that preventable medical errors might cost the U.S. economy as much as $1 trillion each year in lost human potential and contributions, an estimate much higher than patients' direct medical expenses, whether they died or lived.

A 2013 article by James in the *Journal of Patient Safety* suggested that preventable hospital medical errors had become the country's third leading cause of death, after heart disease and cancer—an estimated 440,000 hospital patients died each year from preventable errors. In a transparent system, actual numbers would likely be much higher.

On July 17, 2014, a U.S. Senate Subcommittee on Primary Health and Aging declared that "medical harm in this country is a major cause of suffering, disability, and death, as well as a huge financial cost to our Nation" (U.S. Senate, 2014, para. 12), and that hospitals had been too slow to make improvements. Peter Pronovost, MD, PhD, FCCM, of Johns Hopkins University, testifying at the hearing, reported that although there had been some progress, thousands of patients were still dying unnecessarily from infections, preventable blood clots, adverse drug events, falls, overexposure to medical radiation, and diagnostic errors.

The Senate hearing referenced other reports concerning the impact of medical errors on segments of America's patient population:

- A 2010 Department of Health and Human Services report that stated 180,000 Medicare patients die each year from preventable hospital adverse events

- A 2011 finding by the Centers for Disease Control and Prevention, which estimated that 722,000 patients in U.S. acute care hospitals acquired an infection (1 in 25), resulting in at least 75,000 deaths that year (Magill et al., 2014)

In addition to patients who die from hospital errors, thousands more suffer serious complications from such errors. Preventable medical errors are expensive, both in human suffering and dollars spent. The Senate hearing estimated the financial cost of injury and death due to such errors to be in the billions of dollars each year (U.S. Senate, 2014).

American hospitals need to declare war on preventable adverse events. Yet how can hospitals accomplish this when, as I believe, the simplest practices—like good handwashing—are often ignored or poorly performed, thus increasing the patient's risk for infection (O'Connor, 2011)? Or when, as happened to me, patients and their families are kept in the dark and not told about the preventable errors that caused injury or possibly death to them or a loved one? Or when, as I experienced, hospitals remain silent, failing to take responsibility for or even acknowledge—much less apologize for—avoidable errors that are committed in environments where fear of financial loss often supersedes the patient's or family's right to know?

I believe it will be difficult, if not impossible, for hospitals to shift from a paradigm of corporate interest and financial health to one that makes patient safety the highest priority; as long as a hospital's money engine runs the system, patient safety may be compromised without anyone ever knowing.

Every day, innocent patients are unknowingly pitted against the power and secrecy of a healthcare system run by the hospitals, insurance companies, and, largely, doctors. Most hospital patients who were victims of preventable hospital medical errors continue to be further victimized within a system that encourages silence by the responsible parties, contributing to ignorance and complicity in a system most people mistakenly believe to be better than it is. Financially, it is in the best interest of hospitals to maintain their code of silence.

I went into a hospital for healing and came out more wounded than before. I believe it is incorrect, even foolish, to trust that doctors and nurses will necessarily honor our safety and well-being at all times. Inasmuch as we can be advocates for our healthcare services, we need to be proactive and skeptical—and question and verify what is happening to us. Assumptions are often unconscious. Fear impedes critical thinking. Anxiety narrows perspective.

Sadly, it can be difficult, if not impossible, to be our own patient advocate in a place where we are surrendering ourselves to the safekeeping of mostly strangers at a time when we are vulnerable, hurting, and afraid. Even if a trusted family member is present, that person may not have the knowledge and fortitude to oversee his or her loved one's care, to ask the right questions, and to go up the chain of command, especially when the nurse is unable to perform as advocate. So, where does that leave suffering patients? What are we to do?

Having lain in a bed dying, existing in a coma on a ventilator, suffering from psychosis, living in bewildered confusion inside a broken body and wounded spirit—tended to by many nurses, doctors, aides, and students—I know firsthand how it feels to be powerless, hopeless, and fearful in a hospital: to be betrayed by the very professionals who are supposed to heal you, to be seen as an object or task to be handled, instead of a suffering individual who needs compassionate care. I used to take care of patients like me.

Inside a huge medical center, my life as a patient was centered in my psyche; I sensed whether a caregiver viewed me as a body to handle or as an individual whose body was broken. It was the exception when someone saw me as a real person who was suffering and alone. Long after I left the hospital, I learned that while I was in the SICU, everyone had referred to me as "the patient in Room 2." Since official room numbers were too long to use, staff referred to patients by their room order along the hall—the patient in Room 2, the patient in Room 11, and so on. The following year, as I awaited my bus on a cold winter evening after teaching my ethics class, I struck up a conversation with a young woman dressed in scrubs who was waiting for the same bus. I asked if she was a nursing student. "Oh no," she replied, "I'm a nurse." When I asked where she worked, she said, "in the surgical ICU." Suddenly, before I could identify myself as having been a patient on that unit, she exclaimed, "Oh, you're the patient in Room 2!" A few weeks later, while she and I were again waiting for the bus, another nurse approached us at the bus stop. The first nurse called out, "Hey, this is the patient in Room 2!" Then the new nurse came up to look at me and exclaimed, "I took care of you for 2 weeks!" She did not recognize me awake and without my tubes and machines. That is how I began to think of myself as the patient in Room 2.

As a nurse and teacher—and as the patient in Room 2—I felt compelled to write this book, to use my story to shine light on hospital dangers and a broken system that needs to be drastically improved. Even though I taught and worked in various hospitals before I became a patient, I had no idea that preventable medical errors happened so frequently or that hospitals often value money over truth-telling.

It is impossible to know how many preventable medical errors occur, because deaths caused by medical errors are unmeasured. Talking about preventing such errors takes place in confidential hospital meetings where only those in attendance hear the details. In their 2016 analysis of medical errors, Martin Makary and Michael Daniel, both from the Surgical Department of Johns Hopkins University School of Medicine, explain how the Centers for Disease Control and Prevention compiles the annual list of the most common causes of death:

> The list is created using death certificates filled out by physicians, funeral directors, medical examiners, and coroners. However, a major limitation of the death certificate is that it relies on assigning an International Classification of Disease (ICD) code to the cause of death. As a result, causes of death not associated with an ICD code, such as human and system factors, are not captured. The science of safety has matured to describe how communication breakdowns, diagnostic errors, poor judgment, and inadequate skill can directly result in patient harm and death (p. 1).

The authors outline three strategies to reduce deaths from medical care:

1. Make errors more visible when they occur so their effects can be intercepted.

2. Have remedies at hand to rescue patients.

3. Make errors less frequent by following principles that take human limitations into account.

Makary and Daniel also write that, when death results from medical error, "both the physiological cause of the death and the related problem with delivery of care should be captured" (p. 2).

It is my hope that this book will enlighten readers and lead to greater awareness of what happens in hospitals—so they can protect themselves before becoming patients.

–Donna Helen Crisp, JD, MSN, RN, PMHCNS-BC

DO YOU HAVE A STORY?

Do you have a story of surviving preventable medical errors or adverse medical events? Or do you know someone affected by, or who died from, medical errors or adverse medical events? If so, please send the story to Donna Helen Crisp at thepatientinroom2@gmail.com.

PROVENANCE

"The true beginning of our end"
–A Midsummer Night's Dream, Act 5, Scene 1

My first memory is of utter terror, pervasive and absolute. I am certain of my fate. I am going to die. I cannot move. I cannot speak. I do not know who I am or where I am, just that I am going to die. I am filled with an inexplicable knowing that I will soon cease to exist.

I cannot move; I cannot understand the concept of moving. I am lying in a bed, but I do not presently understand what a bed is. I do not know what has happened to me, nor do I have a notion of what "me" is. I cannot comprehend anything except that I am going to end. There is nothing I can do to stay alive.

I do not know I have been on a ventilator. That I have had five surgeries. That I have been septic and unconscious for 3 weeks. I do not know there are tubes down my throat that prevent me from uttering a sound.

I am unaware of the huge hole in my belly that is hooked up with tubing to a draining device on the floor. I cannot see the monitors that show my heart rate and blood pressure. I do not know what room or building or city I am in.

From a primal, visceral place, I sense my destruction is imminent. Maybe "they" will kill me or maybe it will just happen, my death. I am infused with a terrifying sense of the end of me, whoever "me" is.

At times, I believe I am lying under a coffee table. Up above, on the next floor, I can hear people walking around and talking cheerfully as though they are at a party. Apparently they are going to kill me. Their laughter seems incongruous with my dire situation. How odd to be killed by lighthearted people I cannot see and have never met.

I have no sense of time. My entire existence is in the now, compressed into an inert body totally dependent on the attendance of others. I have no physical pain, no sense of needing to urinate or defecate. I have no hunger, no fatigue, no memory, no future, no sense of body parts or tubes or needles going into me. I have only this fleeting moment, but I am unable to examine it.

It is very strange to be completely without movement. There is no muscle I can move in my entire body. I do not know if my eyes are open. I have no concept of eyes.

"What's past is prologue"
—*The Tempest*, Act 2, Scene 1

Nearly 2 years after my medical nightmare began, I found myself driving back to the place where I had nearly died, where my parents met, where their children earned numerous degrees, where my father died after being brain-dead from complications he suffered after receiving an experimental defibrillator. To the hallowed place where I became a nurse and then nursing professor, and where I now hoped to learn the truth about how a hysterectomy to remove my cancerous uterus became a near-death journey to regain my life and health.

My attorneys were with me as I walked down a long back hallway into the oldest part of the hospital, near the surgical floor where my body was mutilated and disabled. We passed the hospital blood bank, and I briefly reminisced about my final semester in nursing school when I retrieved blood for a young man whose leg had been crushed in a motorcycle accident, whose pulmonary embolism *I* discovered while administering his transfusion on a trauma floor.

We followed a convoluted path of unmarked doors and hallways to a location so sequestered it required a page of written instructions to locate. We entered a small conference room with uncomfortable cast-off furniture, where these seemingly covert conversations would not penetrate the institutional wall of silence.

We have come, finally and hopefully, to get the facts we have not uncovered on our own. To learn what is missing from my medical chart, to hear the truth not yet told to me by my attending surgeon, to receive the facts not yet revealed to the independent experts who scrutinized my medical records. We have promised the hospital administrators we seek no legal remedies, no financial awards. We will not sue. All we want is to understand how my 23-hour outpatient surgical stay turned into five surgeries, a month in the hospital, and years of rehabilitation and recovery. After my not dying, truth is the only reward I seek.

This old building is familiar to me. At one time it was a dormitory for patients from nearby communities who came for chemotherapy, a place where I once visited a patient with a radium implant in her belly, put there to kill her cancer. I remember ignoring the triangular-shaped warning sign on the door as I entered the room and stood right next to her bed while talking with her. I wonder silently if my uterine cancer had begun at that bedside.

I think further back, to the 1960s, when I spent a weekend with a childhood friend who lived here when it was a nursing dormitory. On a quiet Sunday afternoon, she took me to a nearby location, to a room filled with sacks of body pieces soaked in formaldehyde, so I could view corpses used by medical students to learn about anatomy. I still remember realizing those body parts were remnants of people who once lived, human beings who had once had their own foibles and disappointments, hopes and dreams. Did they ever imagine their bodies would be cut apart by students training to become doctors? I still remember the smell of that pickled sanctuary.

My whole life is connected to this place. From this dingy conference room to the whole complex of buildings. From before I was born to the room in that nearby hospital building where I almost died 2 years ago—in the room that ultimately became the site of my reawakening, as my nurse began weaning me off drugs so I could come off the ventilator. There, finally conscious for the first time in weeks, I began to wonder: *How did I get here? What happened? What will become of me?*

"Something wicked this way comes"
–Macbeth, Act 4, Scene 1

The year I got cancer, 1,141 other women in my state received the same diagnosis of uterine endometrial cancer (State Center for Health Statistics, 2010). The American Cancer Society (2016) estimates that in 2016, 60,050 women in the United States will be diagnosed with uterine endometrial cancer. Of them, 10,470 are expected to die. Uterine cancer is the sixth most common cause of cancer death among American women, most typically diagnosed in postmenopausal women at age 60.

I had never known anyone with uterine cancer, nor had I studied it in nursing school. It was only because the faint bloody spots on my panties had recently increased in frequency that I mentioned it to a colleague, a nurse practitioner in women's health. She insisted I needed a biopsy to rule out uterine cancer, so I immediately made the first appointment I could get.

A few weeks later, as my gynecologist pried open my cervix to scrape cells from my uterus, the pain was so intense I had to squeeze her assistant's hand to keep from screaming. My doctor calmly apologized for hurting me, explaining she needed a good biopsy sample to rule out cancer. Ironically, it was the most physically painful part of what was to come. When she called me at work a few days later, I felt myself shift into despair as she gave me the devastating news.

But I did not fall apart until I got home, where I could wail without anyone hearing me. I lay sobbing on my bed, filled with sorrow, and cried long and hard. Remembering that suffering is universal and that I was just one tiny part of humanity helped me feel connected and compassionate and lessened my grief that day. It was a long time before I would cry like that again.

My feelings were so intense that afternoon, I knew I would never be the same—though I had no way to know it would not be cancer that would offer me a premature death sentence. I never imagined that in a few weeks, instead of coming home the day after surgery to snuggle up with my dog in my own fresh, clean bed, I would instead lie in a dark netherworld limbo, senseless and unaware, until I returned to a broken life with no idea how to put it back together.

"The slings and arrows of outrageous fortune"
–Hamlet, Act 3, Scene 1

Cancer is in the details. For me, this meant tiny spots of blood so seemingly inconsequential as to be unworthy of recognition; yet those little dots of faint pink were harbingers of my doom and presaged what was coming for me in late summer. At the time of diagnosis, I had no concept my life was about to be irrevocably changed by something far worse than cancer. Had I known my fate, I would never have consented to the surgery on that particular day.

My diagnosis left me frightened, and I took no time to consider my course. I would fight and hope to prevail. I would not wish for death like my mother had 2 months earlier, when she learned she had advanced breast cancer and saw it as her ticket out of a wretched body and suffering spirit. For me, the news of cancer was shattering, but there was no hesitation; I wanted to stay alive. So I chose a surgeon and began the business of getting well. Although I had an intrinsic fear of new doctors cutting on me, I did not allow myself to think much about the fact that it was summer, the time when new doctors often begin new rotations. I tried not to think about the risks posed by new surgeons, even though I believed inexperienced surgeons would likely be part of my surgery.

A life changes in an instant, for better or worse. I remember once seeing a horrific car wreck on the interstate while hearing emergency vehicles screaming down the highway. Inside the blackened vehicle, still smoldering, dead bodies were waiting for retrieval, bodies of people who moments before were sipping coffee as they maneuvered through traffic, like they did every morning on their way to work. Only a few seconds separated their bodies from other drivers who lived that day because they were far enough ahead or behind the crush of metal and death.

CHAPTER 2

WHOSE BODY IS IT?

"Our bodies are our gardens"
–Othello, Act 1, Scene 3

As a young woman, 20 years before I went to nursing school, I learned to stay away from doctors unless absolutely necessary. Any illusion I had about their benevolence and wisdom was shattered after visiting a gynecologist for a routine pap and pelvic exam so I could get a prescription for birth control pills. In the middle of the pelvic exam, the physician asked me if I was married, and when I said no, he chastised me for having sex outside of marriage. As the exam progressed, he said I had polyps on my cervix and he needed to remove them. With no discussion of, or explanation for, what he was about to do, he called a nurse to assist him as he prepared to perform an impromptu cauterization of my cervix.

I was too surprised and self-conscious, too young and insecure, to stop him for at least a few questions. I lay there, an object draped in white, unable to see below. As he began to stick an instrument into my vagina, he "accidentally" burned my groin. I heard myself scream as I felt the sudden heat searing my tissue. I could smell my burned flesh, but there was utter silence in the room. The doctor never spoke, nor did his nurse say a word. My burned skin was never mentioned or treated.

Eventually, I learned it was common for a woman on birth control pills to have cervical polyps, which were usually benign, and that good medical practice seldom indicated burning away the tissue. If anything, removing such a polyp should have necessitated a biopsy, which was not done.

Amazed more by the doctor's silence than my unexpected pain, I was too stunned and naïve to know what to say, so I said nothing. Later, I wrote him a letter admonishing him for his callousness and lack of respect. He never responded to my letter. Little did I realize his disregard of me was not uncommon. As many people who work in healthcare will attest, many doctors willingly welcome the reverence often bestowed on the position when it is given and even expect it when it is not. Some lose their sense of humility along their professional way. Unfortunately, when doctors become blinded by the power associated with their medical role, they often no longer see the person inside their patients' bodies. Then, they diagnose and treat a body part, not a human being who needs help. Such a tradition has not eroded easily. It still exists among physicians, men and women, and is even more entrenched among surgeons, who seldom know their patients well outside of the anesthetized surgical state.

Even today, some doctors willingly take dominion over their patients' bodies if permitted, allowing little opportunity for questions. It is an old-fashioned approach, from a time when doctors were thought of as holy vessels of mysterious expertise, seldom to be questioned. Of course, there are many doctors who do not practice in this way. Today, there are many doctors who wisely seek and appreciate shared decision-making with their patients, understanding that each patient has a unique perspective on quality of life. Better for doctor and patient to work in tandem than in a hierarchy. Excellent doctors understand this kind of partnership.

"You taught me the language"
−*The Tempest*, Act 1, Scene 2

Two months before my cancer diagnosis, my 82-year-old mother learned she had advanced Stage 3 breast cancer and became a hospice patient soon thereafter. Her tumor had spread into at least four lymph nodes in her right armpit before it was diagnosed. Mother was unimpressed with cancer. For years, she had suffered from numerous health problems, including spinal stenosis, osteoarthritis, emphysema, hypertension, alcohol abuse, depression, and chronic pain. She had not wanted to have the mammogram or the biopsy, much less meet with an oncologist. Because she did not wish to live any longer, she made it clear to everyone that she certainly had no interest in cancer treatment.

Mother's primary care physician told her she would die, if not from cancer, then perhaps from a heart attack, stroke, or something else. She already understood this. Then he described how breast cancer might advance to her brain and cause seizures, with or without treatment. Yet, somehow, he still thought mother might benefit from radiation to shrink and slow down her cancer—even though it would mean radiation treatments 4 or 5 days a week for several months. There would be numerous tests, including computerized tomography (CT) scans of her head, abdomen, liver, and lungs, to monitor where the cancer had metastasized, though he admitted that micro metastases—extremely small numbers of malignant cancer cells— would not show up on these scans. Mother already had little energy. Surely radiation would leave her with none at all.

Mother listened and then made clear she would not obsess about her cancer, or talk or think about it anymore, or have the radiation. I was relieved. I knew that with her advanced emphysema, radiation would significantly lower what little quality of life she still had. Most importantly, she would lose her wonderful hospice nurse who told her she could not have hospice care while undergoing radiation treatment, which meant mother would no longer have help with pain management.

After she refused treatment, I received a call from the supervising physician, who insisted Mother should get the radiation. He did not know her. He did not seem to care that experts recommended against radiation to the chest for someone with advanced lung disease. He did not seem to consider that radiation would increase mother's already high level of mental anguish and physical suffering. He apparently gave no thought to the fact that her hospice care would immediately end when she began making daily trips to the hospital. When I politely explained that radiation to the chest was not indicated for someone with advanced emphysema, he lashed out, wanting to know if I had ever seen someone with open oozing breast abscesses.

I felt his attempt to convince me that Mother should choose radiation illustrated the tendency for healthcare providers to lose sight of a patient's quality of life in end-of-life care. Since he had never met Mother, he easily objectified her, thinking only of her body part—her right breast. I did not want to think he could be motivated by money. Yet, I could not understand why he was so insistent that Mother should undergo radiation treatment, at her age and disease state. How much money would his medical practice gain if the radiation gave mother a few extra weeks or months of her wretched life? Was there financial gain at stake, or could he only see things through the lens of Western medicine's curative philosophy, which tends to greatly emphasize "cure" over "care"? Mother died the following summer, a year after I was in the hospital. During her final months, she received great care from her family as well as her nurses.

"Out damned spot out"
–Macbeth, Act 5, Scene 1

My cancer diagnosis immediately changed my life. One moment I felt fine and in the next moment I was dying. How odd to realize that, as I had watched my mother suffer bodily insults, including cancer, over recent months, my own deadly cells had been quietly multiplying inside me. I never imagined I too was on a journey to death.

There were signs. After reaching menopause a few years back, I had ignored the occasional faint spots of blood in my panties and on toilet tissue during the last two years, thinking these occasional drops were homage to 40 years of full-fledged bleeding. Perhaps my body did not want to completely stop its decades-old habit, and, after all, I still had a uterus, barely used. What difference did a few spots of blood make? How could something so simple and slight be so threatening? And I had no pain, so I ignored it.

As a nurse, I knew the body's universe contains many mysteries. Like everyone, I had a body with quirks, idiosyncrasies usually best left alone, especially because small discrepancies from time to time appear and eventually leave body and memory. My body kept its secret from me for a good long while.

CHAPTER 3

THE SURGERY

*"What fates impose,
that men must needs abide;
it boots not to resist
both wind and tide"*
–Henry VI, Part III, Act 4, Scene 3

Several weeks after my diagnosis, I met the attending surgeon who would be in charge of my case. His well-cultivated pleasantry did not mask his perennial state of hurriedness at my pre-op appointment. After performing a quick exam, he pronounced my uterus was correctly positioned to be removed via laparoscopic surgery, which he would do using tiny cuts and holes instead of one large incision. He said this surgical approach would mean less pain and a shortened recovery period, which sounded good to me since I hoped to miss only 1 week of work. There would be just a few tiny holes in my otherwise perfect belly that would need to heal.

We did not discuss the possible benefits of having a traditional hysterectomy through an abdominal incision. I later learned, from an expert nurse who took care of women whose surgeries had gone wrong, that neither she nor most of her colleagues would ever consider having a laparoscopic hysterectomy. She had seen too many errors, too many lacerations; it was just too risky, she said. She also explained that many surgeons honored a weight factor for laparoscopic surgery, typically using the procedure with patients who weighed no more than 75 kilograms (165 pounds). Although I weighed a little more than this number, my surgeon never discussed body size as a factor in choosing between a traditional incision and laparoscopic surgery, and I did not know to ask.

Nor did my surgeon disclose other risk factors, such as age, or my never having used replacement hormones after menopause. He did not mention how undiagnosed cardiovascular disease can cause sudden heart damage during the operation. He did not discuss the potential risk for large vessel tearing. He did not explain that the major risk of laparoscopic surgery is perforation of the bowel, a condition so serious it can lead to death if the body is not repaired quickly. He did not say that laparoscopic technique can increase the risk of cancer cells spreading between the membranes that separated my abdominal organs from my abdominal wall, something I still think about to this day.

The only thing I told him was that I had a high tolerance for pain, thinking it might prove clinically important, but I could tell he was not listening, wanting to get on with his day. He had already answered basic questions about the surgery, and it was time for him to move on.

I was one of thousands of women he had talked with over his career. As he hurried through the interview, was he thinking I would be a good specimen for one of his new surgeons to practice on, to cultivate dexterity while inserting long instruments through tiny openings into my flesh? After he left the room, one of his new gynecologic oncology fellows, who was to assist with my surgery the following week, reviewed the consent form with me. I watched her write, under *Description of the operation or procedure:* "Possible laparotomy, risks include bleeding, infection and damage to surrounding organs." These words frightened me. But I signed anyway.

She was kind and unhurried with me, probably knowing how scary it all was. I told myself I could trust her—that I was glad she would be working with my attending surgeon. Unfortunately, she was not present at my surgery. A new male fellow replaced her the following week, as I lay on the operating table in an anesthetized surgical coma. So many times I have imagined a better outcome, if only the woman who explained the consent form had done my surgery instead of the man.

"They stumble that run fast"
–Romeo and Juliet, Act 2, Scene 3

I was afraid to have less experienced doctors in a teaching hospital care for me, but I rationalized that they were smart and honorable people striving for excellence under the guidance of experts. Having worked in hospitals, I knew things did not always go well. Nevertheless, I had signed the consent to treat, understanding that I could not have surgery without it, and I was in a hurry to get rid of the cancer.

What I did not know was how many hospital patients die, not because of disease or trauma, but because of preventable medical errors. I believed attending doctors were always working alongside the people they were training. I thought hospital administration and staff always put the good of patients above all else. I was unaware of how detrimental poor clinical judgment and oversight could be.

Later, I realized my fear of new surgeons practicing on me was well founded, and my false belief that trainees would not be allowed to harm me was a rationalization to contain my dread. Fear skewed my judgment. My hurry to surgery, coupled with my inability to deeply consider alternatives, was a tragic mistake. If I had gone elsewhere, to an operating room with seasoned practitioners minus fledgling doctors learning their craft, my outcome would likely have been successful. If I could have waited a few more months to have surgery, when the new summer doctors and surgeons had more experience, I might have had just one surgery.

I believe more medical errors and adverse events occur in teaching hospitals than in nonteaching hospitals. In a 2013 *AARP* article (Kirchheimer), readers were advised to stay out of hospitals in July, given the so-called "July Effect," because that is when new graduates—interns, residents, nurses, and other healthcare workers—usually start their first jobs in our nation's hospitals; this relates to when quality of hospital care plummets, and medical errors increase, during the following month. *My first surgery was in August.*

A study, published in 2011 (Young et al.) in the *Annals of Internal Medicine*, reviewed data from 39 previous studies and found death rates increased 4% to 12% during July and that patients endured longer stays and more time in July due to rookie doctors coming in to replace the more experienced ones leaving. *The new surgical fellow who operated on me had just arrived.*

Fear can clutch a person's spirit so tightly that discernment falls away. Fear can cloud common sense and slant one's course toward tragedy. My critical mistake was deciding too quickly. Fueled by fright, I did not take enough time to consider my course of action. For a long time, I felt some responsibility for my tragedy.

"A dagger of the mind, a false creation"
–Macbeth, Act 2, Scene 1

As I mentioned, my surgery took place in late summer, the traditional time frame for when new doctors and surgeons come into the hospital as the more experienced ones move on to other locations, when clinical expertise drops and fewer doctors are familiar with the hospital. In a 2013 survey (Mattar et al.) assessing the readiness of general surgery graduate trainees for entering surgical subspecialty fellowships, the authors found that 21% to 66% were not well prepared for the operating room, were unable to demonstrate ownership of patient care, and could not operate for 30 unsupervised hours in a major procedure. Further, regarding laparoscopic skills, 24% to 56% were unable to independently remove a gallbladder, atraumatically manipulate tissue, identify anatomical planes, suture, describe therapeutic options, or recognize early signs of complications.

Because my surgery took place in a teaching hospital, the consent form I signed did not mention or portray the extent and significance of how involved new doctors and surgeons might be in my surgery and care. I was only verbally informed that my attending surgeon would be assisted by a new fellow, and that a medical student might be present. Even so, I understood I was consenting for new surgeons to practice on me.

I questioned my attending surgeon if I would be safe while unconscious. He assured me that new doctors and surgeons have been trained to practice safely, either independently or with the assistance of a mentor, adding that he would be right there to aid and assist whomever he might be training, such as the new fellow who participated. He said I should not worry.

Patients cannot have surgery unless they sign the hospital's consent form, or as I call it, a *deformed consent* form. Whether or not patients understand the nuances of informed consent, they are signing and thereby agreeing that, yes, there are potential risks to surgery, as indeed there are. But the hospital controls the form's legality, knowing the patient is implicitly agreeing to accept bad outcomes without fully understanding what that might involve.

Also, patients are often too anxious to consider a worst-case scenario, especially when they do not understand how surgeons are trained. Nor do patients consider the reality of unintended or unforeseen events. Often, patients enter a hospital hoping for the best, not thinking about what might go wrong. Dealing with fear around their surgery may be all they can handle at the time.

Patients are told that a teaching hospital is where the best and brightest doctors work, where experts practice medicine and surgery at the highest level while also training new doctors. Who would not want to be cared for in such an exciting, high-level clinical environment, often considered superior to a small community hospital off the beaten path? Patients are told they will receive the latest therapy and treatment in a place where no matter what happens, there will be someone to take good care of them. Besides, who thinks they will suffer severe consequences, possibly death, as a result of hospital infection or surgical error? But, of course, it happens to someone, at least 440,000 patients each year, according to a 2013 estimate (James). Fancier technology does not mean better patient care. People operate the technology.

If a surgeon makes a medical error during the operation, was it foreseen or intentional? Probably not. But what if, in addition to being unforeseen and unintentional, the error was preventable? Hospitals well understand the language of these consent forms. Their attorneys and risk managers carefully craft the language to minimize any chance a patient may have to successfully argue for legal redress, and they are primarily used to protect the hospital, not the patient.

The following year, I sat in a hospital meeting, listening to an attending doctor scoff that people wrongly assume he is more involved in a patient's care than he really is. That just because he was an attending doctor did not mean he was right there during surgery. For example, he said, he might be in an entirely different building while the new surgeon is operating, or he might only come in to inspect the patient's incision after surgery is over. Listening to his flippant remarks was painful, even though it came as no surprise, not after what I had been through. I sat in silence, grateful for confirmation of what I already knew to be true: Doctors are mere mortals, no better and no worse than the general public. The truly excellent are few, the mediocre are common, and the truly bad are rare. Who would not want to have an excellent doctor?

In my experience, this teaching hospital culture possessed an air of arrogance. The doctors seemed to run the show. It seemed like the hospital and doctors set the expectation that patients had a role to play in training new doctors; that being practiced on came with the territory of having surgery; and that because patients were ultimately cared for by experts (the attending doctors), the risks patients took to support the training of new doctors were worth taking.

Patients who suffer harm or die from surgery will likely never know if they received careless, ignorant, or unsupervised care, or if their outcome was a tragic mishap that could have been prevented. Seldom do operating-room players divulge the errors they make or observe. An institutional culture of blame discourages individuals from speaking up; many fear retribution. A literature review (Okuyama, Wagner, & Bijnen, 2014) of 26 studies revealed that healthcare professionals often hesitate to speak up for patient safety for a number of reasons, including fear of conflict, fear of how others will respond, and concerns over appearing incompetent.

Doctors will say the patient was told what he or she needed to know, including the risks. But, I doubt any doctor has ever told a patient that the surgeon is new to the procedure and might screw up, or that the patient must agree to anything that happens, even if it causes death. Instead, the surgeon will say the patient came to him, needing help, and agreed with what was explained. Again, I doubt many doctors tell patients about the high rate of medical errors in hospitals. Why would they? It would not be in the patient's best interest to know. It would just upset the patient, who is already anxious, and doctors have to learn somewhere. Sick patients need to believe the highest good will be maintained by doctors and surgeons, even in a teaching hospital. Largely, like me, they believe their attending surgeon will be right there to make sure the new surgeon does no harm.

If patients do not want to be practiced on in a teaching hospital, they can go elsewhere. But what if no other area hospital will take their case? What if their medical problem is too complex or unusual for an average hospital? A student once told me her amazing story about when she had experimental surgery at a world-renowned hospital. The surgeon just walked out of the operating arena in the middle of surgery and never came back. Later, the attending doctor told her parents that the surgeon got scared and did not know how to go on, so he left.

I once attended a meeting of mostly physicians who discussed a case study in which a dying, comatose, 85-year-old woman's body was used by dozens of new doctors to practice performing a pelvic exam. The patient's family had not been informed, so there was no consent for these repeated bedside intrusions. The doctors who performed the pelvic exams apparently saw no harm, rationalizing she would never know. The meeting focused on the dying aspect of the comatose woman, not her body being used by students. Listening to the discussion in the room, I felt sadness for the lack of dignity for this woman and anger for the lack of moral soundness. I wondered, did students practice pelvic exams on me while I was in the hospital for a month? After all, I was either anesthetized or in a coma most of the time.

I was already familiar with the long-standing tradition of medical students learning how to do pelvic exams on anesthetized women, though I had not heard about using a woman in a coma. Later, I researched the topic of performing pelvic exams on unsuspecting women who do not give permission and never know what happened to them. Apparently, there is a long tradition for this learning opportunity among medical students, though medical ethics takes a different perspective (Schniederjan & Donovan, 2005).

Hearing about these women brought up a painful memory from my final weeks in nursing school, when I was sent into an ICU to learn how to start an IV on a dying man who was in a coma. He was not on a ventilator. He was orange-colored and near death. I felt uncomfortable because I had never performed this skill, and I knew I would probably hurt him when I attempted to insert the needle into his arm. But my instructor insisted I had to perform this procedure in order to pass clinical, adding that he was too far gone to feel anything. This experience upset me.

In the years since my patient experiences, as I have researched and written this book, I have noticed an increase in public awareness about potential threats to patient safety, as evidenced by patient safety articles in newspapers and magazines; complete books about the topic; and reports on television and other forms of media, including websites and blogs. When asked, I recommend that patients have a friend or family member with them at all times, if possible, to serve as patient advocate and protector. Ideally, such a person would act as a witness to what is happening, identify who comes into the room to do what, make sure that the prescribed medicine is given correctly and the intravenous (IV) line is working (not beeping), assure that adequate pain medicine is available and effective, and so on. But an advocate cannot see inside your body or go with you into the operating arena to watch a surgery or procedure.

"Woe, destruction, ruin, and decay"
–Richard II, Act 3, Scene 2

The morning after my surgery, nine unattended recent medical school graduates checked on me regularly, making entries in my chart nearly every 30 minutes, including such entries as "regular diet" and "discharge to home." The entries stopped as the day wore on and I continued to writhe in agony despite my high tolerance for pain. Had my attending surgeon even remembered my self-reported high pain tolerance, it would not have mattered, because he was somewhere else—at an off-site clinic in another part of the state—leaving the recent graduates to practice on an actual living human being with no one to guide them.

Two years later, the hospital administrators admitted (without apology) that there was no documentation of anyone being in charge of me or the residents the day after my surgery, nor was there any explanation for why no progress notes were written in my chart as the day wore on. If these new doctors had compassion for me, it was displaced by their inability to critically consider what they might not know about my body or the impact of my surgery. They did not appear to question their conceptions and expectations about my clinical picture. With no one to shepherd them, none of these doctors focused on the primary risk for laparoscopic surgery—perforation—for which intense abdominal pain is a major symptom. Otherwise, they might have been thinking, *What if her pain is not just from gas? What if her bowel is torn?*

Because carbon dioxide gas had been introduced into my abdominal cavity to facilitate the use of laparoscopic instruments, the new doctors apparently attributed the cause of my acute pain to be related to postsurgical gas pain, a symptom that is not uncommon postoperatively. However, they also believed my vital signs were not significant enough to consider anything beyond their gas pain theory. If they had, they might have started to critically consider whether my intestine might be torn.

Although I was awake and communicative that day, my physical torment combined with my subsequent coma wiped out my memory, so I have no idea what I was thinking or trying to explain. Did I tell anyone it took a lot of pain for me to reach agony? Did I beg someone to help me? A friend who was at my side during the ordeal later said she did not know what to do. I doubt she realized no one was in charge of the residents.

Now I look back on that day when I was in such danger and wonder, what if the residents had been directed by a wise and competent doctor or surgeon to order a CT scan early in the day, if for no other reason than to rule out the possibility of a life-threatening perforation? What if early detection had been followed by a successful bowel repair, done correctly from start to finish? What if I had awakened that afternoon, sore and relieved, looking forward to going home in a couple of days? Where was the teaching in this teaching hospital?

CHAPTER 4

AND SO, THINGS FALL APART

"To die and go we know not where"
–Measure for Measure, Act 3, Scene 1

During my hospital stay, I traded one cancerous uterus for five surgeries, at least two of them botched, thus setting me on a journey toward death. Memory left me on the day I was admitted and did not return for 3 weeks. The following account is what I have been able to piece together about what happened to me from my medical records as well as what people have told me.

> **August 28, Tuesday, 9:30 a.m., first surgery:** Caucasian female with a history of postmenopausal vaginal bleeding, diagnosed with Grade 2 endometrioid adenocarcinoma of the uterine corpus.

After surgeons cut tiny holes to insert instruments and a camera inside my belly, they harvested lymph nodes from around my aorta and abdominal cavity. Next, they performed a laparoscopic hysterectomy, removing my uterus, ovaries, and cervix, noting, "No disease outside the uterus" and "Complications: None." After postoperative care, I was sent to a regular room to spend the night before discharge the next morning. No one yet knew my surgeons had applied too much pressure as they clamped down on my small intestine with graspers, ironically described as nontraumatic. No one yet realized they had injured my bowel tissue when they pulled it aside to harvest lymph nodes.

Tuesday night/early Wednesday morning: A friend who spent the night with me in the hospital said that I began to complain of agonizing, unremitting pain in the early morning hours, unlike the postsurgery pain I had Tuesday evening. Looking back, I realized my pain ramped up when my small intestine finally burst open, in the exact two places where the graspers had been ratcheted down.

Into daylight hours, I continued to have "stabbing crampy pain, not well controlled by IV meds." My pain was "inordinate for procedure, inconsistent with level of surgery." Incredibly, the inexperienced doctors did not seem to appreciate the importance of physical assessment nor understand that acute pathology cannot be evaluated with just lab numbers. Instead, they relied on the science of numbers while I, the patient, was left almost completely out of the clinical equation. There was no documentation of anyone examining my abdomen.

August 29, Wednesday morning: 17 orders and progress notes were written in my chart over an 8-hour time frame, by nine different doctors, sometimes contradicting observations, orders, and plans of others. My attending surgeon wrote nothing because he was not there. No one took his place. No one supervised my care.

Someone wrote "release in pm if stable, discharge home today or tomorrow." Someone else noted I continued to suffer "multiple abdominal complaints." My early morning vital signs had shown increased pulse and respirations. By late morning, my oxygen level had dropped to 92% (normal is 95%–100%), and my pulse had reached 120 beats per minute (bpm) (normal is 50–100 bpm).

For pain control, I was on morphine, an opiate, and a central nervous system (CNS) depressant. The CNS consists of the brain and spinal cord. Morphine acts directly on the CNS to decrease the feeling of pain. Morphine may lower blood pressure and heart rate as well as slow breathing. Thus, it is important to administer enough morphine for adequate pain control without giving too much that might cause respiratory depression.

The residents did not know or remember, or were not instructed, that abdominal surgery includes a known life-threatening risk for bowel perforation. The new doctors saw my blood pressure as normal, failing to consider how morphine might affect vital signs, with the potential to diminish respiration rate and blood pressure and to mask pain. A good nursing student would have understood that morphine alters the severity and presentation of pain. An attending surgeon in charge of these newbies would have understood as well.

No one appreciated that an average blood pressure does not automatically negate a self-report of excruciating pain. Or that pain should be respected as the fifth vital sign and properly assessed in the patient's full clinical context, along with temperature, blood pressure, heart rate, and respiratory rate. Or that lab values, vital sign statistics, and pain alone do not rule out a torn bowel. Or that, if there is any possibility of a ruptured intestine, the patient needs a CT scan immediately.

> **Wednesday afternoon:** An X-ray of my abdomen was ordered: "Reason: Abdominal pain, rule out obstruction." Presumably, this paved the way for someone to finally order, at 6 p.m., a CT scan of my abdomen and pelvis, but it was not performed until the next day.

> **Wednesday, 8:00 p.m.:** My blood pressure was going up and my breathing was more labored. My oxygen saturation measured 91% on 2 liters of supplemental oxygen and 89% on room air. A normal oxygen saturation level is above 95%. My sister arrived from Arizona to find me in terrible pain. She later told me I said things like, "This is really painful. It shouldn't hurt this bad. I cannot go home like this." The nurse from my first night in the hospital, Susan, had recognized that my persistent and worsening pain was disproportionate to what was expected after my surgery. Suspecting I had a perforated bowel,

she made me NPO (nothing by mouth) in case I went back to surgery. When she came back on for her Wednesday shift, Susan was not surprised to see that a CT scan had been ordered. Once the radiopaque contrast dye medicine was ordered for the scan, Susan brought me the first quart of the disgusting liquid, which I had to drink through a straw. This contrast medium liquid contains iodine, which blocks X-rays from passing through the body, so a radiologist can see where a patient's internal organs might be damaged. It is the only definitive way to rule out perforation, unless the surgeon recognizes it when it occurs.

Wednesday, 10:00 p.m.: Susan brought me another quart of dye to drink. Somehow, with my sister and friend cheering me on, I managed to drink another 32 ounces. By 11 p.m., I was still waiting for transport to take me downstairs for the scan. Almost 10 hours had passed since someone first documented I might have a torn bowel. When transport failed to arrive, Susan and my friend took me with my IV pole to another part of the hospital. At the testing area, I then had to wait until after midnight for the CT scan, which was finally conducted at approximately 12:30 a.m. on Thursday, 40 hours after my bowel had been damaged.

It should never take 12 hours to get a CT scan for a patient if a bowel perforation is suspected. This injury can kill you. It is a medical emergency, in which time is of the essence.

August 30, Thursday, 1:20 a.m.: CT scan results were called to a doctor: "Free intra-peritoneal spill of oral contrast material concerning for bowel perforation. Patient continues to complain of abdominal pain." An hour later, my attending surgeon called my sister to explain I needed emergency surgery, stating that my abdominal pain was poorly controlled despite use of morphine and the volume percentage of my red blood cells had dropped.

It should not have taken almost 2 hours after my CT scan revealed a torn bowel for someone to notify my sister and schedule emergency surgery.

"Defer no time, delays have dangerous ends"
–Henry VI, Part I, Act 3, Scene 3

Once the doctors realized deadly bowel toxins were leaking into my body, they knew I was at risk for peritonitis, an infection of the membrane lining the inner abdominal wall that covers the inner organs. They rushed me to emergency surgery, 14 hours after someone first suspected I might have a perforated bowel.

> **Thursday, 2:54 a.m., second surgery:** After being anesthetized, surgeons cut me open and found two torn places in my small intestine. They performed a small bowel resection, cutting out 4 inches of damaged intestine, then rejoined the new ends (*anastomosis*). Next, they copiously irrigated (washed out) my stomach, hoping to remove all infection. Lastly, they closed the *fascia* (connective tissue) over my stomach muscles, leaving the skin open so they could pack and cover the surgical wound with Betadine gauze.

As surgeons were repairing my bowel, they were unaware the student nurse anesthetist had botched the intubation by performing the wrong technique when he placed a tube down into my trachea. He used a technique known as a normal sequence induction, one that is typically used on patients who have had nothing by mouth (NPO) for 12 hours. The student failed to apply the correct pressure on the *cricoid* (ring-shaped cartilage of the larynx), which allowed my stomach contents (containing toxic dye used in the CT scan) to back up and infiltrate my lungs.

Amazingly, the student nurse did not know my emergency surgery was for repair of a perforated bowel, or that the gallon of toxic liquid I drank earlier was beginning to destroy my lungs. Experts later told my attorney that the induction should have been either by *rapid sequence* (to reduce the risk of aspiration) or with a nasogastric (NG) tube in place to allow for the emptying of my stomach contents prior to the intubation.

According to what my attending surgeon later told me, it took half an hour before the surgery team realized anything was wrong. Since they did not understand I had aspirated at the beginning of surgery, it was only when my pH level (concentration of hydrogen) began to drop that they knew something was not right; instead of being in the normal range of 7.35 to 7.45, my pH level was 7.12.

Regurgitating the CT dye from my stomach into my lungs at the beginning of the surgery caused significant injury to my lungs, which caused me to develop respiratory acidosis, a condition of low pH level. I was going into shock. My injured lungs were failing to remove sufficient carbon dioxide (CO_2) from my body, which meant there was too much acid (CO_2) in my body, which in turn caused my bodily fluids to decrease. I was given sodium bicarbonate and increased hydration to try to increase my pH level. I was developing a life-threatening blood infection (sepsis). Surgery was making me worse. Unconscious and out of the fray, I continued spiraling downward.

You do not need an expert to confirm that communication was poor. The surgeons knew why they were there, but apparently neither the nurse anesthetist (certified registered nurse anesthetist/CRNA) supervising the student, nor the attending anesthesiologist, if present, comprehended my dire situation. It takes experience to achieve the delicate skill of applying the proper amount of cricoid pressure to block the esophagus just enough to keep stomach contents from backing up into the airway. The student nurse had not yet mastered this skill and should not have been allowed to perform it on me.

When people aspirate contrast dye into their trachea and airway, the result may be serious pulmonary complications, including pulmonary edema, pneumonitis, or death. In my case, I suffered aspiration pneumonia, chemical burns to my lungs, and acute respiratory distress syndrome (ARDS), a life-threatening condition where fluid replaces oxygen in the air sacs. I could not breathe on my own. I needed a ventilator. After I was taken to the intensive care unit following surgery, my attending surgeon explained to my family that I had aspirated during the repair surgery. What he did not know to tell them was how badly my lungs had been injured.

Two years later, an expert nurse anesthetist whom my attorney had requested to review my medical records wrote:

> "The surgery was an emergency surgery at 2:30 a.m. The communication was poor. They performed a 'normal sequence induction' with you, something no one would have intentionally done, knowing you'd drunk barium or knowing you had a perforated bowel. This meant they bagged you, pumped in oxygen, which served to push the toxic contents out into your body. The NG (nasogastric) tube was put down after the intubation because you were aspirating. You may have aspirated at the beginning. Whoever they assembled for this early morning surgery did not realize you had come from a barium CT scan. What should have been done was either, (1) a rapid sequence without air, or, (2) a nasal intubation with you awake and alert so gag reflex could work if needed."

If an experienced physician or nurse anesthetist (CRNA) had used rapid sequence induction, a technique often used to quickly induce unconsciousness while safely managing the airway, I would not have aspirated. Perhaps the student was not allowed to do this type of induction because he was not prepared for the risk it posed. Or, if a tube had been inserted through my nose while I was awake, I would have immediately gagged to signal my stomach contents were coming back up. If the attending anesthesiologist and the experienced CRNA knew I had a perforated bowel and a stomach full of dye, they should not have allowed an inexperienced and unlicensed student to intubate me incorrectly. If they did know my situation, they were negligent by indirectly causing me to aspirate. One of them should have performed the procedure instead of the student.

The expert nurse anesthetist also wrote:

> "The charting was poor. An ICU progress note indicated: 'Pulmonary, possible aspiration with intubation.' A post-op anesthesiology note indicated: '18-gauge nasogastric tube placed post induction and sucked one liter of fluid out of her body.' A surgical resident wrote a note to indicate it was anesthesiology's fault that you aspirated, not his."

There was no documentation by anyone in anesthesiology about my failed intubation. Nothing from the attending anesthesiologist, nor from the licensed nurse anesthetist (CRNA) whose only notation about the anesthesiology component of the surgery was, "No complications." There was no documentation from the student nurse about aspiration, though in the records it is noted that he suctioned a large amount (800–1000 cc) of contrast dye from my stomach after the intubation.

The student nurse anesthetist was unidentified in the documentation; his name was not recorded on the surgery's personnel list, as it should have been. Over the years, I tried several times to learn his name, since it should have been on the operative report, but the hospital could not or would not tell me. I wondered if some of the anesthesiology documentation was made unavailable to me in case I wanted to sue the student, which meant sue the hospital.

Although there is no reference to my aspiration in the anesthesiology's portion of documentation in the medical records I obtained, my aspiration is mentioned in three places:

1. Roughly 7 hours after my second (repair) surgery, in a post-op plan, a new surgeon fellow wrote: "Questionable

aspiration of gastric contents occurred during intubation and she will remain on ventilator support."

2. In an ICU progress note written later that same day by a surgical resident who wrote that it was anesthesiology's fault—not the resident's—that I had aspirated.

3. Almost a month later, in my final discharge summary, a surgeon gave me a "Postoperative Diagnosis of ARDS (Acute Respiratory Distress Syndrome) and aspiration pneumonia," and then wrote: "The patient did have a witnessed episode of aspiration at the time of intubation for her second surgery."

From surgery, I went immediately to the surgical intensive care unit (SICU), where I was put on a ventilator and given antibiotics to treat infections. My lungs were too damaged for me to breathe on my own. My body was not getting enough oxygen and my blood pressure was too low. I developed a fever of 101.

Infection eventually caused my wound to rupture along the surgical site. My lungs filled with fluid, making it difficult for the ventilator to adequately expand my lungs and allow for gas exchange. My white blood cell count continued to rise. My antibiotics were changed. Drains were inserted. Sepsis caused me to develop borderline *abdominal compartment syndrome*, which, when combined with abdominal trauma, reduces blood flow to abdominal organs, thus impairing pulmonary, cardiovascular, renal, and gastrointestinal functions. I was on the verge of multiple organ failure and death.

My temperature remained high. One of my drains grew *coagulase-negative staphylococcus*, a frequent cause of nosocomial (hospital-acquired) bloodstream infection, while another drain grew *gram-negative rods*, deadly bacteria that can cause infections in the lungs, bloodstream, and wounds, as well as meningitis. Resistant to most antibiotics, gram-negative bacteria are super bugs, and include *Klebsiella, Acinetobacter, Pseudomonas aeruginosa, E.coli,* and other less common bacteria. A week after the repair surgery, I was sent back to the OR for a third surgery.

"Oh, that this too too sullied flesh
would melt,
thaw, and resolve itself
into a dew"
–Hamlet, Act 1, Scene 2

September 6, third surgery: Surgeons cut me open and found a "collection of dark yellow fluid in left upper quadrant around the spleen"; they then used instruments to hold the bowel while they inspected it, inch by inch, to see if there were any tears or holes, a technique called "running the bowel." They did not find any "evidence of obstruction or perforation." Then, they placed drains in my belly and pelvis and put antibiotics directly into my abdominal cavity, hoping to "wash out" all of the infection. Knowing I would need more surgery, they left the skin and muscle retracted to each side, then filled the 4" × 6" inch hole in my abdominal cavity with a custom cut sponge, from which fluid continually drained through tubing into a negative pressure wound vacuum machine (wound vac). I was returned to the SICU.

September 7: Even though I was still on a ventilator, my respiratory system began failing. On day 8 after my aspiration, it was undeniable that I had developed a potentially fatal condition known as acute respiratory distress syndrome (ARDS). One study showed that patients who acquire ARDS in an intensive care unit have an overall mortality rate of 48.3% (Kao, Hu, Hsieh, Tsai, & Huang, 2015).

September 8, fourth surgery: My white blood cell count remained elevated, indicating infection, so I was taken back to the OR again. The surgeons examined my bowel and "found it to be mildly swollen, but without evidence of acute injury. Abdominal cavity was irrigated and found to be free of pus or any evidence of active infectious process. An attempt was made to close and reattach the fascia, but it was noted to be tight with swollen small bowel protruding through the incision. The decision was made to leave the fascia open and replace the wound vacuum." (Fascia is connective tissue that covers muscle, bone, nerve, artery, and vein, as well as internal organs including the heart, lungs, brain, and spinal cord.)

I was returned to the SICU. My ventilation status began to improve. My white count remained elevated. I continued to receive antibiotics. The wound vac continued to drain fluid out of my wound.

September 11, fifth surgery: I had my final surgery at that hospital. I was no longer septic. My surgeons put my abdominal cavity back together as best they could. They washed out my pelvis and abdomen, inspected my bowel and found no leaks or perforation, then freed up intestinal adhesions (places where bowel sticks together, especially during infection).

Because infection had eaten away so much tissue, leaving the remaining tissue "under too much tension," they could not sew me up. Instead, they covered my abdominal cavity with AlloDerm, a mesh screen made of human cadaver skin minus living cells. The living cells are taken out of this product in order to leave only the collagen, which is the body's main structural protein and is found in connective tissue throughout the body. AlloDerm is like an empty shell placed inside the patient's body so the patient's own blood vessels and tissue can be incorporated into the screen (shell). I have been told that eventually the mesh screen becomes so much a part of your body that it is no longer distinguishable as something that was added. Next, they reapplied the wound vac to a custom-fitted sponge inside the hole in my stomach, then sealed the dressing and tubing so the machine could continue to drain. I would use this wound vac until November 26. My hole did not finally close until March 17 of the following year. My abdominal muscles remained retracted to each side for more than a year, with only paper-thin scar tissue covering my bulging intestines.

After the fifth surgery, back to the SICU I went. My blood cultures showed no new growth of infection. I stopped having temperature spikes. My white count improved. The infections were retreating. I began receiving medicine for high blood pressure. On September 13, I received two final units of blood. The wound vac dressing was changed every 48 hours. I was still in a medically induced coma and on a ventilator.

The pre- and postoperative diagnosis for my final surgery was, "fascial separation, *iatrogenic*, following intra-abdominal sepsis. Wound vac." Iatrogenic refers to the adverse conditions a patient suffers when a physician (or other provider) inadvertently causes harm to the patient, by medical treatment or by diagnostic procedures. Apparently, my attending surgeon had accepted that, except for endometrial cancer, my medical problems stemmed from a perforated bowel and a failed intubation, both of which were avoidable. While I likely suffered other iatrogenic harm I never knew about, I know for sure that doctors caused the following:

- Surgeons tore my small intestine in two places without knowing it.

- Doctors failed to provide me with adequate postoperative care.

- Doctors failed to provide me with continuity of care.

- Doctors failed to diagnose my injured bowel in a timely fashion.

- Doctors were late in ordering an abdominal X-ray.

- Doctors were late in ordering a CT scan of my abdominal cavity.

- Surgeons were late in repairing my bowel after perforation was confirmed.

- Anesthesiology allowed an inexperienced student to intubate me incorrectly.

- Anesthesiology caused my aspiration after I consumed a gallon of dye.

- Anesthesiology was unaware of or failed to acknowledge my aspiration.

- Anesthesiology caused me to suffer life-threatening complications to my lungs.

An anesthesiologist who fails to sufficiently comprehend a patient's history for potential complications during a surgery may be committing malpractice before the surgery even begins.

"I am to wait, though waiting so be hell"
—"Sonnet 58"

While I was enduring my iatrogenic nightmare, my family was living their parallel version of my tragedy. Two of my sisters had planned to visit me at home the morning after what should have been a short, successful surgery. However, as my condition worsened and I was rushed to emergency surgery for a bowel repair, they came to the hospital later that morning to see me in the SICU. My surgeon told them the surgery had not gone well; there had been a problem when I was intubated for the surgery to repair my intestine. He informed them that I was very ill and that I aspirated when I was intubated. My sisters were stunned to see me full of tubes, in a coma, clearly dying.

Over the following weeks, one or both of my sisters came to the hospital each day to learn of my changing status. Later, one sister remarked about how much focus was placed on the numbers. She said she did not realize medicine was all math. Each day, they would attend to me in any way they could. They played music, as though it might serenade me away from death. They helped bathe me, when a nurse suggested it would be therapeutic for them to lay hands on me. Another sister, far away in Montana, prayed with American Indians in a healing ceremony for my survival. As for me, I was in a coma; I was somewhere else.

My mother remained alone in her house in a nearby city, slowly spiraling into dementia. She could not understand what had happened to me, though she knew I was sick. She longed to see me. One rainy day, one of my sisters brought her to the SICU and later described the visit to me: When Mother saw me, her oldest child, lying helpless and lifeless, she cried as she held my hand and gently spoke to me, as though I was still her baby.

With few exceptions, friends, relatives, and colleagues who wanted to see me were discouraged from visiting. Knowing I was a private person, my sisters knew I would not like people staring at me while I struggled to stay alive, unaware of my surroundings, unable to comprehend my situation.

As my saga continued week after week, my sisters monitored my daily progress and kept others informed. One sister knew I was having problems with my gut and lungs. She told me years later that, because she understood the lymphatic system helped maintain fluid balance, filter blood, and aid in the body's immune response, she had asked a doctor how my lymphatic system was being affected by infection and shock. She was stunned when he responded by sarcastically asking if she was a doctor. He stated that it was a teaching hospital, and if she did not like the way my case was handled, she could take me to a different hospital.

In the SICU, I continued to fall prey to uncontrollable events and lack of accountability, while my sisters, equally powerless, focused on my medical care and survival. Beyond that, they could not comprehend how my 23-hour outpatient surgical stay had become weeks of suffering in an intensive care unit, on a ventilator, while having to undergo five surgeries. They suffered with the stress that I might die, inside an institution that, in my case, failed to support families of comatose patients.

CHAPTER 5

FIGHTING TO HOLD ON

"A wretched soul, bruised with adversity"
–The Comedy of Errors, Act 2, Scene 1

Within an hour of entering the hospital in late August, my memory stopped. For 3 weeks, dozens of people watched over, looked after, and ministered to me, but "I" was gone, without awareness to know what was happening. As people came and went, doing things to my body and watching me, "I" did not exist. There would never be any way to recollect those missing weeks. My chemically comatose, bloated body had separated from my soul.

I remember checking in at the registration desk and handing over my insurance card and identification to a nonmedical young man. I was surprised to feel tears spilling down my cheeks. My anticipation of coming to the hospital for surgery was suddenly an overwhelming reality. The sadness of the moment felt crushing. The admitting clerk did not know what to say, and I felt sorry for making him uncomfortable.

Next, I remember walking down a hallway to a small room where I changed clothes and waited with a friend who would stay with me after surgery, through the night, and then take me back home the following morning. Soon, an anesthesiologist came in to ask me a few questions. The OR was ahead of schedule, and my surgery would start around 9:30 a.m. My memory ended in that little room.

"A sorrowful soul"
–*Love's Labour's Lost*, Act 5, Scene 2

As I lay in the SICU, septic and on a ventilator, cancer was no longer an issue; it was infection that threatened my life. It took a team of people to keep me alive: nurses to oversee the tubes entering my mouth, throat, nose, neck, hands, belly, and urethra; a respiratory therapist to manage my ventilator; and a nutritionist to monitor liquid food being pumped into my stomach.

Because aspiration had introduced the radiographic contrast dye into my lungs, causing severe damage, my body could not get enough oxygen. My flooded lungs caused my blood vessels to dilate, which caused my blood pressure to fall dangerously low. The intravenous fluids I needed to keep my heart pumping caused me to blow up like a water balloon. I became a huge weighted sponge, filled to over-flowing. I was expected to die.

My heart was still working, but I was weeping fluids. Much of this excess fluid traveled into my abdominal cavity, where three Jackson-Pratt (JP) drains were surgically implanted. Every few hours some-one emptied and measured the fluid that came out of these drains. Over time the fluid turned from pink to light yellow to clear.

A ventilator continued to breathe for me, which required me to re-main sedated, in a medical coma, so I would not struggle to breathe on my own. Blue tubes connected the ventilator to an endotracheal tube (ET tube), which passed down the back of my throat into both branches of my trachea, so the ventilator could push air into my sick lungs.

The fluid, which was necessary to keep my circulatory volume ade-quate and my heart pumping, created complications. Secretions with nowhere to go continually accumulated at the base of my lungs. The

ET tube prevented me from coughing up this fluid. When I tried to cough, an alarm would sound and someone would run into my room to thread a suction catheter down through the ET tube into my lungs to vacuum out the secretions. Along with secretions, the suctioning removed air, causing me to gag. When I became conscious enough to sense something was being stuffed down my throat, I would gasp in panic, while trying to reach up to protect myself from invasion. My hands were tied to the bedrails as a preventive measure, and strong white tape had been applied to my face and around to the back of my neck to keep the tube in place. Each morning, I was rolled over and onto a hard board for a chest X-ray to monitor the fluid accumulation in my lungs.

I was helpless in this battle of failing lungs. When I could not breathe and my gasping became more intense, I was given medicine to sedate me back into unconsciousness, to an unremembered world where I was no longer in hell, where I could breathe over a bank of violets and watch tiny sweet flowers wave in the sun.

In addition to the ET tube, a nasogastric (NG) tube ran through my nose, down my throat, and into my stomach, creating a fluid highway, running most of the time with liquid food that needed little digestive effort. Since I could not swallow, medications were liquefied and pushed down into my stomach with a syringe. Before procedures, nurses reversed the flow of this tubing and quickly suctioned everything out so fluids would not get into my lungs when I was laid flat.

IV lines were stitched into each side of my neck. On the right side was a large bore catheter, a central line with three ports, entering a subclavian vein. One port measured the vein's pressure while the other two ports were for medications too caustic to the smaller veins in my arms. Often, I had six different medications infusing into me at one time. On the left side, an IV line entered my jugular vein to serve as a backup in case I needed immediate transfusion of blood or fluids.

Stitched into an artery in my left wrist was a radial line, which enabled continuous blood pressure monitoring. It was also used as access for nurses to collect blood samples from a port without subjecting me to the discomfort of repeated needle sticks. Every 12 hours, my blood was collected and tested for oxygen content and chemical analysis.

Between my legs was a silicone Foley catheter, which passed through my urethra and into my bladder to drain urine into a bag. On each leg was an inflatable compression sleeve which intermittently applied pressure to prevent blood clots, for which immobile patients are at high risk. Once formed, blood clots can travel to major vessels in the heart, lungs, or brain, possibly causing a stroke or heart attack and perhaps even death.

There was a 4" x 6" hole in the middle of my belly, and my abdominal muscles remained retracted to each side. Because infection had eaten away the skin, there was no way to sew up the hole. As long as there was a hole, the muscles could not be put back in place.

Because of concern that infection might continue to plague me if the wound did not properly heal from the inside out, a wound vac machine remained in place. Every 2 days, a new piece of black foam was custom fit into the hole from which a tube drained fluid into a machine on the floor. Alarms sounded if something went wrong. On the day I was to leave the unit for another part of the hospital, I finally saw this sponge. It looked like it had been wrapped in a dried sheet of seaweed, or nori, which is used for making sushi. (I have always hated sushi.)

After I got home from the hospital, I continued to need the wound vac machine 24 hours a day for 2 more months. I vividly remember November 26, the day the tubing was finally removed. After 3 months, I could finally take a shower. As soon as I got home from seeing the doctor, I stood in the shower and cried as hot water streamed down my face and torso. It was Thanksgiving time, and I was grateful for the simple gift of these sensations.

Although the machine was gone, I still had a small hole in my belly, which required me to do daily wound care until it finally closed on St. Patrick's Day of the following year. I considered painting a four-leaf clover over the area to signify my good luck in being alive.

"What's done is done"
–Macbeth, Act 3, Scene 2

After receiving fentanyl for pain and Versed for sedation for weeks in order to remain on the ventilator, it became increasingly apparent that I was experiencing a paradoxical reaction to the Versed. Instead of calming me, it was causing extreme agitation. I was not clearing it out of my system.

Versed (midazolam) is a short-acting minor tranquilizer used in surgery and other procedures for sedation and to relax muscles. In my case, it was used for amnesia, to keep me suspended from reality, in another dimension and without memory. Sometimes patients suffer unintended reactions to this medicine, such as anxiety and agitation.

Fentanyl, sometimes called synthetic heroin, is a narcotic analgesic, a hundred times more potent than morphine. It is often given in conjunction with a benzodiazepine, such as Versed. The withdrawal from fentanyl is associated with nervousness, hallucinations, anxiety, depression, and disturbance in understanding or formulating language.

My nurse, Henry, talked with my sisters, and all agreed to stop the medications quickly, in an attempt to limit the length of my discomfort, instead of slowly weaning me off the drugs and thus prolonging my misery and confusion. After 3 weeks in the hospital, I returned to consciousness, only to suffer from psychosis, a mental state in which a person does not understand reality. Psychosis can cause utter terror as well as occasional pleasant out-of-body excursions. I experienced both states.

Delirium, though often undetected, is very common in the intensive care unit (ICU), especially among mechanically ventilated patients. One study of multiple centers found the prevalence of delirium to be 32%. In some specialized units, the prevalence was higher, for example, in a burn unit where a majority (77%) of patients developed delirium. Another study found the incidence of ICU delirium ranged from 45% to 87%, depending on how many of the ICU patients were on a ventilator (Cavallazzi, Saad, & Marik, 2012).

"Cut her out in little stars"
–*Romeo and Juliet*, Act 3, Scene 2

I am free, untethered to flesh and bone, or even to "me." I am not of this earthly domain, nor of this room or building. I see my body below, lying off-center across a bed, while other patients lie still on nearby white-sheeted beds. Nurses move in silence. There are no sounds.

There are no ceilings. I move effortlessly as I watch others in repose. Below me, I see two women biblically washing a woman's hair, gently anointing her long brown strands with handfuls of water from a baptismal font. It is me.

I enter unknown spaces of an adjacent building. I have no thought or apprehension, no pain, no suffering. I am free to luxuriate in my amorphous journey.

I am no longer a body given breath by mechanical lungs. My arms are no longer receptacles for dripping chemicals. I am no longer submerged in temporary annihilation. I am coming back to my life.

Each time, after a few moments of freedom, fear would force me back into my motionless body, into a sensation too unknown and horrible to produce clear thoughts. I could not move or speak or understand the activities and people around me.

Throughout my first day off the ventilator and drugs, my psychosis began to slowly intermingle with reality, as my brain began to process where I was. The more I understood, the stronger my instinct to survive grew. I knew Henry was my protector; he would not harm me. He would help me survive and live. I was right.

CHAPTER 6

LOCKED INSIDE MYSELF

"Then begins a journey in my head"
—"Sonnet 27"

While people viewed the motionless body of a breathing woman, I knew I was alive. I could sense the energy and motivation of people around me. Since I could not move or speak, my invisible faculties became heightened. I could literally feel other people's energy. Some viewed me as a set of skills on their to-do list. Others, through compassionate eyes, saw me as an injured woman in need of care. Occasionally, I heard a man on a loudspeaker giving cheerful updates about special products in a department store. I thought his name was Dr. Fine. I could tell he was kind. Although I never saw or spoke to him, I believed he would help me go home. Later, I learned he was a ward clerk who sometimes used the intercom to communicate with staff. He was not a medical person, and his name was not Dr. Fine.

I saw a young boy sitting on a blue throne near the nursing station. He was a small Japanese emperor, a boy king, dressed in embroidered, royal blue silk clothes, wearing an elaborate blue headdress. It was his birthday; he was 4 years old. On a nearby counter were various celebratory foods, bowls of treats and cups of soda to joyfully commemorate his life. His mother was a nurse on the unit. I wondered how she could do her job and also watch over her young child. But there he sat, dutifully, quietly, politely, without fuss, like a little Buddha, amid the daily confusion of a place where people clung to life and sometimes slipped into oblivion. Later, I learned it was monthly staff appreciation day, with snacks and beverages on the counter, so staff could easily partake throughout their busy day. There was no royal child.

I heard a noise outside my only window and believed it was a car driving around steep curves, up a mountain road. This happened over and over, until I could almost see an Italian sports car traversing the sharp terrain, on its way to some interesting destination. Two years later, I looked through this window and saw the red brick wall of a facing hospital wing a few feet away. The noise I had heard was from a machine, not a car.

I saw a group of motorcycle hippies walking to and from a room next to mine. One of them wore a shirt that said, "Hells Angels for Jesus." Later, I learned they were visiting a friend who was badly hurt in a motorcycle accident. He did not survive.

I heard a strange repetitive noise coming from a nearby curtained room. It was intrusive and unsettling, sounding like a siren. I thought the patient must be in bad trouble. Later, I learned it was the sound of a door opening and closing.

I heard two women softly talking outside my room late one night. I listened to every word, as though they were on the radio, while they shared archetypal stories about coworkers, family, food, men, and relationships. Their quiet conversation comforted me, as I realized in amusement they had no idea I could hear every word they were saying. Later, I learned they were housekeepers.

One night I had a new nurse. He was initially friendly, but for some reason I did not trust him. I began to wonder if he was diverting pain medicine for his own use. He would come to my bedside holding prefilled needles and then put them in his pocket, giving me nothing. One time, he curtly asked me if I was hungry, thirsty, or in pain. I somehow indicated "No," since I could not talk. He gruffly replied that there was nothing he could do for me in that case and abruptly left. Throughout the long night, I hoped he would not come back, even though I was lonely and craved someone to be with me. Later I wondered if he had medications for other patients. Eventually, I communicated with the unit manager about his unkindness. Even though my body was in havoc, my instincts were sharper than usual, and I knew he was not a good nurse. Ultimately, he was dismissed.

"Oh God, that one might read the book of fate"
—Henry IV, Part II, Act 3, Scene 1

Personal history prepared me for the uncertainty and lonely hours in the SICU after my coma. I had long practiced mindfulness, to reach what I called the refuge of the holy moment, a place with no past or future. Before the tubes came out and I could speak, there was much to observe, both in my room and in my head. But when my thinking took over, my strongest thought was about the future. I had to go home.

A troubled childhood turned me into a determined and persistent young woman, my resilience firmly embedded. I was accustomed to accomplishing my goals. At 15, I became a lifeguard. In college, I published a short story in a literary journal, hoping to impress my in-tellectual boyfriend. After serving on jury duty, I went to law school and earned a juris doctor. When I was 30, I drove across the country to Los Angeles, where I performed as a singer-songwriter and pianist on the nightly open-mic music circuit for 2 years.

I came back east and worked as a French teacher and a waitress. Then I went to nursing school, working full-time and commuting to school to earn two degrees. It took 7 years. After I became board-certified in my specialty, I chose nursing roles with significant chal-lenges. Ultimately, I became a nursing professor. During the weeks between my cancer diagnosis and surgery, I worked tirelessly for hundreds of hours to finish an article based on my graduate-school research. It was published in a journal soon after I came home from the hospital.

I knew how to not give up; my survival instinct was very strong. I was not surprised to wake up from a coma with an unrelenting desire to go home. Tenacity may have saved me. The following year, Henry, my SICU nurse, told me something he found to be true in his nursing experience: Some patients have a fighting spirit, some do not, and that is often the difference between whether they live or die.

My earliest tangible thoughts were, *What happened and how can I get out of here?* I knew I was in a place of death: death by inadvertence, by ignorance, by default; death by a cascade of sad and unwitting actions and decisions. I also knew no attempted murder charge would be brought, no criminal charge argued in a moral court of dignity and human respect. In the next few years, no one would take ownership of the errors that befell me. No one would ever simply say they were sorry for what happened to me. Had this been otherwise, I probably would not have written this book.

In spite of my ferocious will to go home, I had no strength and no voice. I could not talk. I was too weak to hold a pen. I could not move any part of my body except my eyelids. After lying motionless in a bed for weeks, and losing 20 pounds of muscle mass, my body was deconditioned. I was temporarily paralyzed by weakness. Parts of my trunk and legs were numb. Outwardly, I had to give up any decision-making. I had no other choice.

My earliest memory in the SICU was my (false) belief that if I sat in a chair long enough, my doctors would see I was strong enough to go home. Henry and I communicated, without words, and he helped me get into a chair, where I sat for several hours to prove I could leave. It did not work. I was not yet thinking clearly.

My doctors could not hear my silent pleas. I remained alone in my inner sanctum of brain and spirit. My full-time task was to pay attention. While others exerted their external powers, I was my own vigilant sentinel, watching and remembering what people did to me.

*"We know what we are,
but know not what we may become"*
–Hamlet, Act 4, Scene 5

I am an amnesiac with no pre-existing life, my slate wiped clean by drugs. I have no awareness there has ever been a slate. I am paralyzed; I can hear the ticking thoughts inside my frozen body. I am a prisoner, captured and immobilized. My only freedom is deep and silent within.

I am virginal to the world, without history, without self-reflection. I am a young child, wounded in spirit, suffering without being able to understand why. I am demented, lost in the unfathomable deep, inside inescapable confusion, in a sponge where nothing stays, spiraling into nonexistence inside a living death.

I am completely alone, connected to no one, not even myself. I am submerged to the human core, in a place no one can reach. I am a labyrinth of endless pathways, riding connections of neural firing inside fantasy and imagination, submerged into singularity, completely separate from the rest of the universe.

I am in holy retreat, in reverent devotion to the sanctity of the eternal now. There is no past or future.

CHAPTER 7

RETURNING FROM THE VOID

"When I waked I cried to dream again"
–The Tempest, Act 3, Scene 2

As my senses returned and the psychosis subsided, I began to see and hear again. I had survived. I was alive, but barely. The only memories I would ever have of the SICU were from my last weekend there, after I was taken off the ventilator.

That Saturday, I had a few visitors. I wondered why I could not talk, unable to feel the tubes in my throat, most of which would be removed the next day. One sister read to me from Alan Alda's memoir. Another sister played a CD of Vedic chanting and Hindi music. I looked at a photo of my dog. I began to notice the sounds of the busy unit outside my room.

Because Henry was off for the weekend, a new nurse, Linda, took care of me. On Saturday morning, when she came in to see me for the first time, I tried to lift my gown so she could see the huge hole in my abdomen, since this was what everyone wanted to see. I thought I was being helpful, but she immediately scolded me to put my gown down and not show my "privates" to people. Her words stunned me.

A little later, she returned and pulled my gown up to inspect my abdomen. Unable to smile, I thought, *I must be alive if I can be amused in spite of my deplorable condition!* She could see only my broken body, so she did what many nurses and doctors do and treated me like an object, a sick object.

After coming off the ventilator, I had tried without success to write. My writing looked like chicken scratch, and I wondered if I had suffered a stroke. Mid-morning, I somehow conveyed to a doctor that I wanted to write something, and he brought me paper and gave me his pen. This was a grand achievement. I needed to document the four reasons I should be allowed to go home, convincing myself that when doctors studied my list they would have no choice but to let me leave the hospital. I began to write, "Number one: Yesterday I sat in a chair for several hours, which proves I am capable of going home." While I no longer remember the other reasons, I vividly recall how convinced I was that my written statement would help me get out of there.

While I carefully wrote, Linda entered my room and immediately swooped in to remove the paper and pen from my hands. I did not need to be doing that, she said, having decided for me. She obviously had other plans for me, and, oh, was my brain ticking away. *That is no way to treat me*, I thought, *Where is your compassion? I am a person who cannot speak, and you have just dismissed me. I am a grown woman, not a child who needs to be reprimanded.*

Everything I had taught my nursing students about understanding, listening, seeing, and caring for patients came to life as I suffered from Linda's foolishness. She saw me as a powerless body to control and manipulate. I had no voice so I did not exist. Only the artful and expert nurses understood "I" was not my body. Henry knew I was present. He never treated me like a child simply because I had no voice.

Strangely, thinking about my cat helped me deal with my hospital situation. A year before, my 13-year-old Maine Coon cat, named Taylor, had his rear leg crushed in some unknown trauma outside. After an orthopedic surgeon reconstructed his leg with pins and rods, Taylor wore a splint for 3 months to prevent him from walking. He had to stay in a spare bedroom with the door closed, alone, away from his brother and the dog, as they might engage him to play. Situated on a pillow next to a tall window that came down to a few inches from the rug, Taylor could watch birds flit about in nearby shrubs and trees. For 3 months, as he lived his solitary life in that small room, he was serene and accepting, never once trying to leave. When the splint was finally removed, he was still required to remain alone at his window for another 6 weeks.

In the hospital, I often remembered how gracefully Taylor had accepted and acclimated to his fate. I thought of him as a supreme being in the universe. I aspired to be like him, though unfortunately I had no birds to watch. Instead, I studied nurses and doctors.

"Tis the mind that makes the body rich"
–The Taming of the Shrew, Act 4, Scene 3

After most of the tubes were removed from my throat on Sunday, I could finally produce raspy words. My world was expanding. I was now an object with an external voice.

Linda was my nurse again, so I resumed my subservience to her direction and command. She was efficient and skilled, and I felt confident in her activities. By the end of her long shift, I could finally speak and I thanked her for her excellent care, which seemed to surprise and please her. I did not take it personally that she had belittled me the previous day. I could see beyond her ingrained behavior and personality to her capable nursing skills and strong work ethic. And I realized that I seemed incapable of holding onto grudges, judgments, or biases. As soon as one formed, it immediately dissolved.

On this same day, nurses helped me stand up between the bed and wall. My deconditioned body seemed to weigh a thousand pounds, 10 thousand pounds. I felt the world spinning around me while dizzying bright hall lights whirled around my body, which felt solid, gargantuan. When I was sat back down, I knew I could not go home. I had absolutely no physical strength. I could not sit or stand or move, much less walk on my own. Once again, I surrendered to my sad hospital fate.

Now that I was more conscious than psychotic, there was much to do in Room 2. I looked out into the busy hallway, which led to the nursing station and doorways of other patient rooms. I eagerly watched people come and go, while trying to understand what they were saying. Otherwise, my mind was preoccupied with food, which I had not eaten for several weeks. I was told I would not be allowed to eat or drink until I passed a swallow test the following day. The test would determine if I could eat and drink without aspirating, after having tubes down my throat for several weeks. Until then, I was content to dream about tomato soup with cheddar cheese, sweet cherry Diet Coke with crushed ice, and so much more.

That evening, I learned one of my nursing students, Jenny, would be working the night shift. As I anticipated her arrival, it was the first time I felt joy since before my cancer diagnosis. When she walked into my room, she filled it with the light of her smile and energy. It made me feel truly happy. In prior days, she had seen me bloated and comatose. Now, I could speak. I asked her questions about the unit, her schoolwork, and the other students. She was sweet and endearing. Everything she said was golden.

Around 4 a.m. on Monday, she told me she was taking her break. Since I could not sleep, I waited for her to come back, visualizing her talking with friends as they shared stories in the night's final hours. I was surprised by the power of my feelings about her, wishing I could be a young, beautiful nursing student taking her break instead of me, inside a broken body. She reminded me of when I was young and whole, with shiny hair and spirited eyes, filled with hope for my unknown future.

Decades earlier, as I was about to finish college, I was in love with a man my father had forbidden me to see. In late November, I eloped on a Tuesday morning, instead of going to biology class. Within weeks, I had graduated and started a new job as a social worker, working with impoverished families and young children. Then, I never considered how sickness and bad luck might alter a life, re-routing and scarring body, disabling heart and hope. I never thought about being older and sick. I never thought about being a nurse, much less a dying patient.

"Food of love"
—*Twelth Night*, Act 1, Scene1

It was a busy Monday morning, my last day in the SICU. But before I could be transferred to another part of the hospital where life-sustaining care was not needed, I had to undergo the swallow test.

Three young women with long golden hair, all perky and smiling, entered my room. They could have passed for actresses in a shampoo commercial, or a medical Charlie's Angels trio. They spoke in unison, using short sentences, as they described the test. Perhaps they used this approach in case a patient had dementia and could understand only a few words at a time.

I could talk, albeit with a scratchy voice, but I said little, as I watched them set up their accouterments: a metal spoon for presenting me with food and liquids, a pipette straw for placing liquid at the back of my mouth, a tongue blade, a suction machine, a glass of water, and ice chips.

The speech pathologist in charge of training the other two women began the test.

After inserting a camera down my throat, she directed me to swallow foods and liquids of varying consistency: blue applesauce, blue cracker, blue milk. The color blue was used since it was not a color normally found in the body. If I swallowed properly, there would be no blue food or blue liquid in my airway. I paid close attention. I very much wanted to pass this test. I was hungry, very hungry. But it was an emotional hunger, not physical. The food in my fantasies had little connection to my actual body. I saw my little blue meal as a medical intervention, not something to sate my appetite. Swallowing those small amounts of food did not seem like eating. I passed their tests and left the SICU late that afternoon. The golden angels represented my gateway to ice chips and beyond.

"What dreams may come"
–Hamlet, Act 3, Scene 1

There is no sound. I am standing over a dead body, which lays flat on a bed, covered with a gray cotton blanket. I place my fingertips on the cloth over the chest and immediately hear air leaving the corpse as it deflates. I push harder and the air leaves faster. I pull back the cover and see my father's mother, Martha, who died in 1982. There is no pillow, her forehead is tilted back, her dead eyes are open, her mouth is pointed upward. I put on gloves before I close her mouth and eyes. I feel no emotion. I wake up.

Death is not necessarily a bad thing. It may mean your worst nightmare has ended and your suffering is over. If I had died in the hospital, it would have been okay with me, for I was already gone. Given the chance, I might have stepped into the abyss, past the point of no return, toward the "shining light" of lore. And, oh, what sweet release it might have been, to be spared all the suffering that was yet to come.

Being in a coma was like being dead, although my respite from life's travails was only temporary. I no longer thought about papers and deadlines, students and exams, lectures and conferences—or of washing dishes and paying bills. I was unaware of the tribulations of world events. I forgot about my mother, who was continuing on her journey of cognitive disintegration, dreaming in the deep about her parents and childhood.

My coma was a reprieve during my near-death surgeries, while I was transferred from stretcher to bed to platform, over and over again—besieged by nurses, technicians, and doctors who cut, manipulated, examined, and treated me. Death would have spared me a future of heartache and struggle. But entering death, after weeks of prolonged medical interventions, was not the way I wanted my life to end.

One day about 10 years before my hospitalization, I was walking my dog in the fading light of an early summer evening when I saw a woman pulling weeds at her mailbox. I stopped to say hello. I remember nothing of our short conversation except for this: Her husband of 48 years had died unexpectedly the year before, on a Sunday night, while they watched *Singing in the Rain*. She had left the room for a few minutes to fix snacks, and when she returned, she saw him slumped over, dead, in his big chair. I told her how sorry I was for her loss. Walking home that evening, I thought about this man I had never met, how lucky he was to have taken his last breath while watching Gene Kelly dance.

"The time is out of joint"
–Hamlet, Act 1, Scene 5

It feels as if life goes by in a second, moving faster and faster the older you get. Time is relative and can bend or lengthen depending on your perspective. A broken heart virtually ensures time will stop, as though sorrow needs all of infinity to feel the pain. Moments of transcendence occur at the speed of light, perhaps because to savor them would end them. Alas, our worst moments seem to last much longer than our happiest ones.

But is there any sense of time in a coma? I think not. There is no perception of time, so there is no time. Life is on hold, so there is no life. Being in a coma is like being dead, with no awareness of the present, no past or future. And if I had gone straight from coma to death, I would never have known that I had experienced a brief interlude of living death before I slipped away forever.

AWAKENING

"Awake dear heart, awake"
—The Tempest, Act 1, Scene 2

Late on a Monday afternoon, after almost 3 weeks in the SICU, I was quickly wheeled down a hallway, onto an elevator, and to another part of the hospital. No amount of longing or attachment to going home could change my ongoing hospitalization. I was still hallucinating at times. Since most of the tubes had been removed from my throat, I could speak a few gravelly words. Although I could not move any part of my body, I was finally beginning to see the true nature of my reality. I had no physical pain to hinder my awareness. Most of the time, I was able to be in each moment. This was the beginning of my transformation.

I did not need to arise at 3 a.m. in a Buddhist temple to do sitting meditation with strangers in a silent, darkened room. Because I could not move, my expensive hospital bed became my sitting sanctuary, where I lived inside my deconditioned body, quiet and still. Peace was now, in the present moment. Fear lived in the future; I wanted no part of that. The past was gone.

My identity now resided in an indefinable space, as big as eternity and as small as my bed. Wrapped, bound, and immobile, I was a living mummy. In or out of the moment, I kept returning to my spiritual heart, the only place I did not feel desolate. I observed my feet covered in a sheet; they looked like two snow-covered peaks. I gazed out my huge window to see only the tinted windows of a side wing.

I was no longer the patient in Room 2. Here and now, the SICU was far away.

Because I could not move my body, I lay in my undulating bed, which continually moved my legs to help prevent blood clots, yet my heart and mind roamed freely. Sometimes I forgot I could not feel my right foot and left thigh, or my entire abdominal and pelvic area, all numb from nerve damage after the five surgeries. I was reminded of Christopher Reeve, the actor who had portrayed Superman in the Hollywood movies. After falling off of a horse, he became paralyzed. Later, he proclaimed he was not his body. I was not my body either.

No longer able to identify with my motionless body, who then was I? My body had been cut apart, over and over again, in the area of my third chakra—the location of the solar plexus, which some people believe is the body's center of life force and power of transformation, in addition to governing digestion and metabolism. I lay awake in my hospital room, alone most of the time, and wondered what injuries I had suffered beyond those of my physical body. Would I have the emotional strength to put my life back together? How did five surgeries affect my body's center of life force?

I could not comprehend the physical significance of my injury because I could not arrange my body and lift my head to see the 4" x 6" hole down below, fitted with a custom-cut medical sponge that was changed every 2 days so it could properly drain fluid into the expensive machine on the floor. My focus was on the weariness of not being able to move any part of my body, especially my legs, and of always having to stay on my back, unless someone placed a pillow under my legs or slightly shifted my carcass toward the side.

While I knew little about the changes in my body, I paid attention to everything outside myself, hearing every swish of the curtain each time someone opened my door and the airflow shifted. I thought of my nearby bedfellows down the hallway, dealing with their own personal crises. Patients seldom came to this women's unit unless something bad happened in an operating room. I would never meet any of these patients, or see their rearranged bodies, or hear about their revised fates. I never left my room, not until the moment I was discharged from the hospital.

"I have not slept one wink"
–Cymbeline, Act 3, Scene 4

Sleep continued to elude me. No matter how many times I closed my eyes, I never lost consciousness. I could only rest. But my body had been resting for weeks. It was my now alert, ticking brain that could not be repressed. After it got dark outside and day staff went home, I was always in the physical position for sleep, prone on my bed, without distractions except for the monkey chatter of my thoughts. Still aware of where I was, still hearing little noises from the hallway, I just could not go to sleep.

Having come out of a coma only a few days before, did I unconsciously associate sleep with death? I imagined other patients throughout the hospital enjoying a temporary respite from suffering while they slept. I longed to do the same. Instead, I did the second best thing I could imagine, I used those quiet night hours to meditate, to practice Vipassana, which in the Buddhist tradition means to have insight into the true nature of reality, to see things as they really are. Sleep time became meditation time.

Except for the mandatory vital-sign ritual or scheduled medications, no one entered my room at night unless I requested them to do so. Dark hours were a long buildup for the next morning, when I longed to receive information to help me understand what had happened to me and how I might be able to move on with my life. While I endured the long nighttime emptiness, I took in the silent nuances of darkness and early morning light, making sure the curtains remained open so I could see the beginning of daybreak.

White sheets and thin blankets covered my skin, which covered my organs and bones. Hard featherless pillows supported my head and shoulders. My muscles offered little support for moving a blanket or a leg. *Later, I learned I had lost 20 pounds of mostly muscle mass.* I was too weak to use any of my limbs and needed assistance to reposition myself or change a pillow.

Inside my body, inside my bed, inside my room, the next moment arrived, then the next one, and the one after that. Though I longed to escape my current tragedy through sleep, I could not sleep. I wondered if my unintended vigilance was to ensure no one would harm me again.

Sometimes I could not grasp where I was, in which hospital or what city. I wondered if I was in a hospital where I used to work, far away. Then I would think hard enough and my location would come back to me.

Sometimes I watched the clock high up on the wall; the bathroom door was left ajar so a slither of light could reveal the clock's numbers to me. Though I tried to decipher what time it was, I found it confusing and wondered why this kind of clock was used in patient rooms.

I never watched television, not after the first and only time someone turned it on, thinking I would enjoy *The Oprah Winfrey Show.* Though I loved Oprah Winfrey, I could not tolerate the bizarrely unreal programming. Eventually, I came to realize the artificial world of television being programmed through a small screen hung high in the room was antithetical to my current powerful meditative state of *now*. It was too distracting; I could not watch. Perhaps the precipice of death had left me incapable of being entertained by what now seemed like overly produced artificial images.

I contemplated the shower stall, just a few feet from my bed. Though I could not turn my head to see into the tiled room, I longed to stand in there and feel hot water streaming through my gnarled hair, down my back and legs, cleansing away my weariness and sorrow. *It would be more than 2 months before I would finally take a shower again.*

I imagined the sounds of my home, the daily talk of wrens and cardinals, a car coming down the street, an early morning truck sounding from a nearby highway, occasional airplanes flying over, wind and rain, cats padding down the hall, a ticking bureau clock, the outside HVAC unit going on and off, the hum of a ceiling fan, the telephone ringing . . .

I lost the month of September. By the time I was discharged, I had not been outside for a month. Summer had fled, taking with it the high temperatures that had baked and dried the earth, killing my St. Theresa hydrangeas. I thought, *Well, I missed some heat and the season's first dead deer lying by the roadside. That's OK.*

"True it is that we have seen better days"
–As You Like It, Act 2, Scene 7

My room was a living tomb. Because I could barely move, I only saw what was in front of me and slightly to each side. I never saw my bathroom, only a few feet away, unless two people helped me move to the portable potty next to the shower. I was alone most of the time, enough time to memorize every detail I could see.

Daylight was for the repetitive details of hospital workers: the radiology technician, the food server, and so on. A young man who rode his X-ray machine like it was a giant scooter arrived early each morning. I called him Clark Kent, after Superman's alter-ego, and began to listen each dawn for the sound of his machine, as he entered the unit and rode down the hall to my room. He was always pleasant, unaware of my tragedy, with no idea how much those little moments of interaction lightened my heart.

Just after dawn, doctors entered my room to view my body on display, another assessment to perform along their journey to truth. It seemed like a hundred different doctors came by throughout the days I was there, as though I was an observational requirement for everyone working in the gynecologic oncology medical lineup. I wondered if some of them just wanted to see what a woman looked like after surviving a 3-week septic coma nightmare in the SICU. I wondered if a memo had gone out requesting them to be nice to me, as though their reassuring smiles would mean I had not almost perished at their hands.

Looking back, I doubt their visits were personal. I was a statistic, a number. Patients were admitted, treated with or without complications, and then discharged, unless they died first. I was an aberration, still in the hospital a month after I was supposed to have left. A middle-aged female with surgical complications who had not died and was thus still in the medical game, with a big hole in her gut, with continually changing numbers to record and analyze, lest the object of science be forgotten.

Each day the smiling housekeeper came in to ritualistically move a mop along the floor and empty the trash container. I tested her one day after she cheerfully asked her routine, "How are you?" I suspected she could not speak English, so, I smiled as I said, "I am frustrated, impatient, irritated, and unhappy." Happily, she replied, "That's good." This amused me. My sense of humor was still with me.

Smiling staff came every day, offering to wash my body and change my gown and sheets. One nursing assistant stood out. She gave me more than pleasant energy; she gave me connection. Sometimes her bright chatter was the best part of my day. Hearing details of her personal life helped me believe I would soon return to the land of the living. Even though I was just one of many women whose bodies she attended, she was truly present with me. Once she mentioned she might go to nursing school, and I offered encouragement. I knew she already had the requisite ingredient to practice the art of nursing, an open heart and loving spirit to see the patient as a whole person.

One afternoon, someone holding a clipboard briskly walked into my room and began to talk in a chipper voice, without introducing herself. She announced that she had come to talk with me about my smoking habit. Smiling at her, I said, "Well, before you begin, there's something you should know. I smoked my last cigarette about 30 years ago." She froze, looking at me while her brain reconfigured. She said she had obviously been given the wrong information and immediately left. I wondered if this little mishap was a common marker of a medical system too big for its own good.

Most of the people with whom I interacted each day did not know or care to know about my situation. They did their jobs. I also did my job. I paid attention to nuances of inflection. I remained poised to hear any new sound, something more than curtains moving or water running. Feeling somewhat detached from my traumatic reality, unable to recall events because of my coma, I sometimes experienced moments of intense anxiety, feeling afraid and helpless after almost dying. After 30 days, acute anxiety becomes post-traumatic stress disorder (PTSD).

When technicians, nurses, nursing assistants, physicians, food workers, nonclinical staff, colleagues, and family entered my room, I was on guard to discern if they would help or hurt me. Were they in a hurry? Were they careless? Inept? Menacing? Did they possess professional expertise? Or were they the rarest kind of person, someone who understood that a sick person is scared, vulnerable, and often capable of sensing the intention and attitude of others?

"Bruised arms hung up for monuments"
–*Richard III*, Act 1, Scene 1

Since I did not sleep, I had a lot of time to think. Sometimes I considered my hands. I never saw them in the SICU; they were tied down until the end of my stay. Now I looked. My fingernails had not grown, which I later learned was due to the trauma I suffered. My skin had an orange hue, which I assumed was also secondary to trauma, as well as malnutrition. One thing I noticed was that my hands did not hurt. Since I had not used them for weeks, my carpal tunnel symptoms had temporarily disappeared.

I thought of my father, a brilliant lawyer whose hands had written thousands of words on long yellow notepads and typed numerous letters and legal briefs on his small manual typewriter. How he had argued not once, but two times, before the U.S. Supreme Court, and I had attended one of those hearings. How he had held too many glasses of liquor and, by my count, at least 600,000 cigarettes to his mouth, which ultimately ruined his heart. Before he died all those years ago, he played golf and piano and gesticulated with each corny joke he told.

My mother had used her hands to take care of her little girls, sewing our clothes, cooking, cleaning, and doing yardwork. She also managed to be active in local politics and theatre. While we were teenagers, she went back to school to earn her doctorate. In the summer after my trauma, a few months before she died, Mother's right hand was so swollen from lymphedema, caused by her advanced breast cancer, that the ring she had worn for half her life was painfully tight. It was her mother's engagement ring, made in Germany in the early 20th century, with a "pure white diamond," as mother liked to say. She had always wanted me to have it. One day she asked me to drive her to a nearby jewelry store to have the ring removed. Since she could hardly walk, the jeweler was kind enough to come out to the car. He gently cut off the ring and handed it to me.

One of my sister's hands was left in a permanent claw position after a man high on crack cocaine broke into her apartment one hot summer night and tried to kill her, streaking her body with a packing knife, severing her ulnar nerve. She lost dexterity in several fingers, making it more challenging to play music. Because of her buoyant energy, no one ever seemed to notice her hands or the scars on her face.

Another sister used her hands to trace muscles, manipulate tendons, and move cranial sacral fluid at the base of her clients' skulls. Another sister used her hands to write poetry, walk dogs, and garden. My youngest sister, born with Down syndrome, had a single palmar line across each hand.

As I lay in bed for 9 days, not sleeping, I thought of all the ways I had used my hands. Playing guitar and piano, kneading bread, typing, making clay bowls, sewing, painting watercolors, gardening, caring for my patients and students, and writing, always writing—essays, short fiction, poetry, columns, and lectures.

CHAPTER 9

BODY AS BACKDROP

"Therein the patient must minister to himself"
–Macbeth, Act 5, Scene 3

My attending surgeon came to see me a few times. He was always smiling. One day I was feeling particularly prickly and had prepared my thoughts ahead of time. Because I already had an advance directive, which did not fully relate to my current situation, I needed to give him an update about my wishes. Advance directives include living wills and healthcare powers of attorney, both of which I had.

He walked over to my bed and I began telling him that, even though I did not know how to get through my current situation, I knew for sure I could not tolerate any new bodily insult. Firmly, I said that if something else happened to me in the hospital, like a stroke or heart attack, I did not want anything else done to me, including surgery or treatment. He smiled and patronizingly offered that many people have some depression when they go through what I had been through.

I did not tell him I was not depressed, that a better description of my emotional state included words like heartbroken, betrayed, determined, sad, afraid, and resolute. I repeated my wish to be spared from further medical interventions. He said I would have to put my intentions in writing, which I did that same day, though in no way did I expect him, or anyone else, to honor my poorly written sentence on a scrap of paper, which I still have. From my own healthcare career, which had focused, in part, on ethical decision-making, I knew that even a person's legally notarized advance directive was sometimes disregarded in the heat of a moment, such as if a family member told the doctor something different from what the patient had indicated. It is hard to have power when you are unconscious.

My attending doctor's sidekick, the new fellow who had participated in my first surgery, visited me a few times. Obviously ignoring the hospital policy against staff wearing scent, he wore cologne so strong I could taste it. Perfunctory in every way, he did not seem to know or care about me as a person. I believed that to him I was just a body he had operated on.

In one visit, he began reprimanding me for having requested in pre-op a month earlier that my nursing students not be allowed to be my hospital caregivers, telling me I did not have the right to make that request. The fact that he was wrong, according to hospital policy, did not surprise me. That he chose to chastise me about this while I lay broken and confused amazed me, given what had happened (at his hands) and how much I was still struggling with the aftermath.

Although my attending surgeon was the top doctor in charge of my case, he rarely appeared. Instead, numerous other doctors came by my room each day. I remember a few. One woman often came before daybreak, staying less than 5 minutes, to perfunctorily place her stethoscope over my heart, a superficial show of patient assessment. She was pleasant and kind. Months later, I saw on the medical billing that she had charged me over $600 for each of these visits. This changed my perception of her kindness.

One day a doctor entered my room for a moment as I was trying to reposition myself. I asked if she could help me and was surprised to see a glint of fear in her eyes as she explained that she did not know how to do anything like that, but she would try. Her expensive medical education had not prepared her to reposition a patient in a hospital bed, something nursing assistants without a high school education can easily do. How well insulated are these doctors who learn their trade, sometimes at their patients' expense, and then stay forever separated from patients. Great doctors are different. They are wise enough to know there is an art to medicine, as well as the science.

A woman I had never met entered my room one morning, with physicians trailing behind her. She explained she was filling in for my attending doctor. When she asked how I was doing, I shared that I had started writing—in my head at the time—a book about my trauma experience. Locked into her power position, she could not seem to connect with me, one human to another, or she would have sensed that my enthusiasm was perhaps a miracle, given what I had been through. She imperviously chided me, telling me I could not do that.

To her, I was an object. To me, she was a diminished human being. I watched her mouth move on a face that appeared to lack the necessary musculature for smiling. I was a patient on her checklist. No doubt she had already made her clinical judgments based on data and was just briefly saying *hello*, never imagining I might provide her with any insight into my condition. When she spoke to me, the light inside the room, and inside of me, dimmed. She will never know how a moment of kindness might have helped me. Perhaps she had been awake all night—no excuse. Perhaps she was in the throes of a divorce—no excuse. Perhaps she had wanted to be a dancer instead of a doctor—no excuse. The Dalai Lama says his religion is kindness. That surgeon, and others like her, would do well to understand the simple meaning and power of that message.

A 4th-year medical student was one of the best doctors who took care of me. She had chosen my floor for her clinical semester rotation because she hoped to eventually become an OB/GYN doctor. Each time she came into my room, she listened to me and earnestly attempted to provide me with some of the information I would need prior to my hospital discharge. She approached me as a person first, subject second. Her grandfather bore the name of a famous literary character. More than once, I joked with her that she had descended from that lineage. She always smiled back at me. I hoped she would never change into a version of the female surgeon who had dismissed my humanity.

"Nurse, come back again"
−*Romeo and Juliet*, Act 1, Scene 3

One night, a new nurse came in to meet me. She was orienting to the unit while shadowing my assigned nurse and informed me she had come from a famous medical center, where she specialized in the care of pregnant drug abusers. She spoke with no hint of warmth, and her projected self-importance seemed an obvious mask for insecurity. Later, when I asked her to page my doctor, she replied in a demeaning tone, asking if I was sure I needed to speak with him, challenging the necessity of my request. I explained this doctor had specifically told me to call him if I wanted to speak with him. She replied that since she was new, she did not know how to page the doctor. I countered if she could not figure out how to call him to let me know and I would do it. Two hours later, when she returned to my room for something else, I asked if she had ever reached my doctor. Her curt reply that she had contacted the doctor made it obvious that she was unhappy with me and would do no more than absolutely required. I reminded her that whether or not she liked me, it was her job, as my nurse, to advocate for me. She glowered at me and left the room without comment.

Her brazen lack of compassion was in stark contrast to my favorite night nurse, Susan, whom I first remember meeting one night when she answered my page around 2 a.m. She explained she had been my nurse weeks ago, on my first and second nights in the hospital, a time erased from my memory. She said that on the night she and my friend took me for my CT scan, she thought my bowel might be perforated. But when she returned to work the next night and did not see me, she figured I must have been discharged. Unbeknownst to her, I was fighting for my life in the SICU. Now, 3 weeks later, I was glad to meet her again.

I explained I might be having a bowel movement but was not sure, because so much of my body was numb. Given the raging infection my body had battled, it was not known how my bowels would function once I became medically stabilized (that is, not actively dying). Susan opened up the sheets and moved aside the pillows to inspect between my legs and confirmed that I indeed had had a bowel movement and reminded me that this was good because it meant that my bowels were working. She gave no hint of disdain as she wiped and cleaned me up.

I sensed she saw me as a temporarily sick woman, someone with wisdom, history, and heart, not a big baby in need of a diaper change. She saw me as a grown woman who would get better. She saw me as a teacher and a nurse.

On the few occasions I saw Susan, she shared stories of her childhood, family, and career while she cared for me. Listening to her, I began to feel like someone more than a body or patient. I began to feel like me again. As her words activated my identity as a person, my pervasive sense of powerlessness began to lessen, and I realized that one day I would be more than a woman in a bed who could not move. I would leave the hospital and return to life.

Her words of normalcy had a profound impact on my wounded heart. She exemplified the ideal communication I had taught my students. *Stay inside each moment with your patient, sharing humanity, connecting as one human being with another.* Susan understood this. She was an expert nurse.

Unfortunately, Susan could not work 24 hours a day. One morning, a wound care nurse hurried into my room to change my abdominal dressing, which required sterile technique. I was to receive IV pain medicine as soon as she arrived, since it would take effect quickly. But this nurse was in such a hurry, she refused to wait a minute or two, and abruptly left. Luckily, I had noticed her unwrap a pair of sterile scissors which she stuffed back in her pocket on her way out of my room. When she returned about 10 minutes later, she pulled the now-contaminated scissors out of her pocket to use on me. "Stop," I said, explaining the scissors were no longer sterile and could not be used, which I am sure she knew. Obviously angry, she opened a new packet and proceeded to change the sponge in my abdominal cavity without speaking to me.

On another day, this same nurse came to help me use the bedside toilet, since I could not stand or walk alone, or wipe my backside. Again, she entered my room in a hurry. She was visibly huffy and angry. She was no underling. I am sure she saw herself as too good to help with such a lowly task, which she had been assigned because of staffing shortages.

She helped me to the bedside toilet. After I peed and wiped my front, without warning, she suddenly tried to yank me off the toilet seat before helping me finish. Terrified I would fall, I yelled out, "Stop!"

I had already met this nurse on the unit and knew she was a recent graduate of the BSN program where I taught. After I realized what kind of nurse she was—a bad one—I was disappointed that someone like her represented the school where I worked. Later, I told the unit manager that the wound care nurse was not a good nurse: She was more interested in having power than helping patients, and she was impatient, impersonal, and dangerous. I announced emphatically that she was not to enter my room again. How many patients have the ability to understand sterile technique or the willingness to request a certain nurse no longer take care of them? Not many.

In addition to Susan, another wonderful nurse, originally from Indonesia, often took care of me during the day. She told me that when she first came to this country to work as a nurse, she was most impressed with prefilled saline syringes, that there was nothing that modern in the village where she used to live. One morning, not long before I left the hospital, she came to my room with tears in her eyes. "I am so sorry. I have too many patients this morning. I need to discharge two of them. I cannot come back to you until later. I cannot do anything for you now." I felt sorry for her and assured her that my sister would help me when she arrived in a few hours. I felt compassion for the angst of my overworked nurse as well as gratitude for her kindness. She cared so much about her patients that she struggled with how to fairly care for all her patients, given her time limitations. Her dilemma was a case study in the ethical concept of justice.

On my last weekend in the hospital, late on Saturday night, I was left in a chair beside my bed for more than 2 hours before someone answered my call to help me into bed. When a nurse finally came, at around 2:30 am, she said there were not enough nurses to help all the patients. The next morning, staffing continued to be critically short. Fortunately, one of my students was working as a nursing assistant on my floor that morning. Although I had vowed to her earlier that I hoped she would never have to do my personal care, when she stopped by to say hello, I told her I had to break my promise. There was no one to help me to the bathroom, and I had been waiting for hours. She smiled and gracefully assured me it would be an honor to help me. Later I learned that she eventually quit her job because of chronic staffing issues. She was often the only nursing assistant on the floor.

"Unbidden guests are often welcomest
when they are gone"
–Henry VI, Part I, Act 2, Scene 2

I was alone much of the time in my quiet room except for occasional visits from a few friends and my sisters. I remember a foot rub, beautiful flowers, a bunch of get-well cards, a friend helping me eat soup. A couple of times, Henry, my savior SICU nurse, came by to say hello on his way home, after working a 12-hour shift.

Some visitors, however, were not so welcome. Aside from a few colleagues who had permission to see me, I firmly requested no visitors.

Nevertheless, my wishes did not deter a couple of faculty members. They seemed determined to satisfy their own needs, ignoring my directive. Coming to see me was about them, not me.

One of these colleagues was heading toward the elevator to my floor one afternoon, when someone reminded her that I did not want visitors. Undaunted, she continued on her way and in a few minutes was in my room. She pulled up a chair to sit and stare at me, I presume to see for herself how terribly sick I was. She expected me to entertain her with certain facts about my harrowing ordeal. I answered her questions, doing my best to reassure her I would survive. Later I worried that she might have used her hospital privileges to inspect my medical record, something forbidden, though not preventable.

Another faculty member came to see me and immediately burst into tears. As she continued to weep, I felt obligated to take care of her. I assured her I was okay, though I was not. She was someone I hardly knew and who, I later learned, was generally unstable. No doubt her tears were about her own pathos and fears, projected onto my situation.

These two people exemplified the reason I had asked for no visitors. People who assume a sick person in a hospital wants visitors might be wrong. The motive to visit a patient may have more to do with making the visitor feel better, rather than the patient. My experience taught me it is best to check with a patient and listen to his or her wishes before deciding whether or not to visit. Those patients who are really sick may have little energy for idle chitchat. Getting well while in the hospital is hard work. And just like any hard work, interruptions can make things even more challenging.

TOLERATING UNCERTAINTY

"Who is it that can tell me who I am"
–King Lear, Act 1, Scene 4

I was awake for nearly all of the last 9 days and nights I spent in the hospital. At first, I could not move, eat, read, or use a telephone. I could not hold a spoon. I could not understand the clock or television. I kept hearing the Italian sports car, which had followed me from the SICU. But I was alive and awake, watching and waiting to see what would happen next.

Early on, I was filled with painful gas that could not be alleviated. Once, for 24 hours, I lay without moving, eyes closed, somehow existing in a suspended state of acute discomfort. I could not swallow medicine that might have helped dispel the gas, because even a sip or two of water made me gag and throw up, even when there was nothing in my stomach. I was surely in a living hell. So I burrowed all the way into the pain.

The resilience I developed in my childhood helped me accept what I could not change in the hospital. Whether walking home from school trying to outpace bullies or waiting for someone to come home and save me from a parent's rage, I learned how to bear anything. I went to college without goals for my future. I chose men who were incapable of loving me. I believed anguish was normal. I believed heartbreak was inevitable.

Although I eventually healed into an authentic individual, I still carried within me a hardened center of unyielding resolve. I could wait forever. Sometimes this was a character flaw, but sometimes it served me well. My resilience allowed me to tolerate the uncertainty of my illness and hospital stay. It was a blessing, because I followed a long and unpredictable road of recovery as I tried to return to the self I was before this ordeal. I faced fear and pain for a very long time.

"Tomorrow creeps in this petty pace from day to day"
–Macbeth, Act 5, Scene 5

I was an expert at waiting: for letters, for lovers, for dreams, for traffic, for morning, for darkness. As a child, I waited to grow up so I could escape home. As an adult, I waited for true love so I could be happy. I waited for my life to happen until I realized waiting was not living.

Day after day in the hospital, waiting was my main job, and because of my lifelong experience with waiting, it was something I could do with grace. It was a mind-set, a way of being. I waited for clarity so I might understand what had gone so terribly wrong. I waited for the truth. I waited to go home.

I was convinced someone would tell me the truth. Surely people were monitoring my recovery. They knew where I was, that I could talk, that I could listen. Any moment, someone would explain and apologize. I was sure of it. Someone would assure me that everyone was so relieved I was alive, especially in the face of my regrettable circumstances. Any minute, someone would knock. For days, I maintained a powerful belief that I would be acknowledged, that someone would say I mattered and how sorry they were. I was wrong.

Each time I heard the door to my room open, I asked myself, *Will this be the moment I find out? Who will tell me? A hospital administrator? A physician? An attorney? Maybe a risk management specialist?* With each passing day, my belief weakened, as I wondered, *Where are they? They should know I am no longer in a coma. I can't believe no one is talking to me yet. They should have already come to see me. Why would they make me wait to understand? This can't be . . .*

At some point, when I was strong enough to hold the phone, I called the hospital from my room to ask for someone to come see me. Now, I cannot recall exactly what I said. But, after a day or two, an old woman, looking to be in her 80s, appeared in my room with a young teenager. She was some sort of volunteer the hospital used for various patient errands. She had no idea why she had been sent. I thanked her and said I did not need anything. Then I gave up and called a woman who I knew was a malpractice attorney. I knew she would help me.

Months later, someone from the hospital told me there had been communication between the SICU and the hospital's public relations and legal department about my case. The SICU was informed that no one was to talk with me about anything that had happened. They were told that I had grounds for a lawsuit against the doctors, and that if staff members talked with me, they might lose their license.

"To be, or not to be, that is the question"
–*Hamlet*, Act 3, Scene 1

Thinking about leaving the hospital made me happy and scared. I knew I would be safer at home, but I was still sick. I could barely move. I had little faith in my body. I worried about my lungs, my abdominal muscles, which were still retracted, and the hole in my gut, which did not close until 6 months later. I worried about the smell of my bodily secretions, the amount of my urine, my low-grade temperature, and my swollen legs. I worried these were messages of doom. I lived in fear of cancer resurrecting itself and stealthily entrenching my bowel, or some unsuspecting new location. When I thought about cancer, I did not feel like a survivor, though I was grateful I did not need radiation or chemotherapy.

Would I be able to handle my future life? What would I do if I could not regain physical strength and resume some normalcy in my life? What if I could no longer work? I lived alone, so who would help me? What would I do with my pets? Would I ever like my body? What if I was destined to endure horrific physical suffering? What if my life would no longer be worth living? Like all fears, mine were about the unknown future. Thankfully, I recognized this and just kept letting go and being here now. And then letting go again and again, over and over. Practicing eternity.

The hole in my body was like a hole in my life that bore through my history, my present, and into my future. While I was dying in the hospital, people went to work, gave birth, bought cars, ate dinner, and went to football games, to movies, to church. News was forever changing. Life went on without me. While I was a prisoner in a bed, watched by technicians and strangers, newspapers piled up at my house. Litter boxes overflowed, mail multiplied, and seasons shifted from the dry heat of summer to the browning and crinkling of leaves preparing to fall.

"Sit you down in gentleness"
—As You Like It, Act 2, Scene 7

I left the hospital with a gritty resolve to survive, although I could not define what that meant with words. I was determined to get beyond my crippled existence.

I suffered as a child from a pervasive darkness of mood, filled with waiting and fantasy. After my sisters and parents went to sleep each night, I had imaginary conversations in my bed with my future husband and children. Only later did I realize I was creating the life I did not have. Normalcy. Connection. Kindness. Love.

I often felt invisible, but despite that, I prevailed. I managed to stave off hopelessness; I cultivated waiting into an art form. I could have won medals. I could have lived on death row, because I could stay inside myself endlessly, avoiding the unknown by concentrating on the now.

Going home, the horrific nature of my predicament left little room for anything but survival. I had to stay in the moment. Not getting ahead of myself, not thinking about my unknown future. I had to remain determined and grounded in survival mode. The future would unfold in its own time. Doubts were traitors.

So, homeward bound I went, with these goals: to somehow survive, live, and move beyond my tragic body situation; and to find out what happened to me in the hospital. I vowed to write a book so that I could share my story with the world. I vowed not to live in a regretful past, but look ahead to the future with hope.

The first thing I did when I entered my home was to use my newly attached elevated toilet seat. I was thrilled to learn I could wipe myself without needing anyone to help me. I also realized that the archaic bedside commode at the hospital had too small an opening for my hand to fit through while seated. I would have fallen on the floor if I had tried. I was thrilled to reclaim this private chore.

HOMECOMING

"Thus bad begins and worse remains behind"
—Hamlet, Act 3, Scene 4

I came home at the end of September. Summer had fled, though its heat continued into October. People were planning for Halloween. A month earlier, I had left for the hospital on a humid August morning, already visualizing being home the next day to cuddle in my comfortable bed with my pets for good company. Neighbors and friends would bring food and wish me well. I would take naps, watch television, eat comfort food, talk to friends on the phone, and open get-well-soon cards. I would take my time to read the morning newspaper, while sitting on my deck to draw strength from nature. I would quickly regain momentum and go back to work the following week. Best of all, I would no longer have cancer, just a sore belly. I could leave crisis mode, let go of my breath and the fear and stress that had occupied my spirit for several weeks. But it was not to be.

After arriving home late in the day, my neighbor came over to help my friend assist me with my walker. I entered through the side room, level with the driveway. I took one formidable, tiny step up into the kitchen, then slowly walked into the open dining and living room area, and down the hallway to my bedroom. With the exception of my office in a little loft above my living room, my entire house was on the ground floor. For this, I was very thankful.

With a person on each side of me, I slowly sat down on the edge of my bed. I was gently helped to twist my torso so I could lie back on pillows while someone lifted up and straightened out my legs. I was exhausted but relieved to be home. I missed my dog, though, as she had been sent to another town for safekeeping. And, although my two aging Maine Coon cats were present, they were no doubt unhappy they had been alone in my house for a month, with only occasional visitors to feed them and clean the litter box.

There was little joy to summon; I was too sick. I could barely think about each moment much less my future. My losses were too overwhelming to contemplate. Survival had used up my energy in the hospital. I knew my body and life were shattered. My prevailing concern was an important one—could I pee by myself? Imprisoned in a body that no longer worked very well, I could barely think much beyond bodily functions.

However difficult life was about to become, at least I was home. If death might take me, I knew it would be easier than what I was facing. I did not know how to reconstruct my life when everything had changed, and I had no idea what came next. Most of us need to feel that we have control over our lives. I had lost that illusion. But I was determined to find the truth. I had an attorney sitting beside my bed 4 days later.

I had lost 20 pounds of muscle weight and could only walk a few steps, and only with assistance. I was still connected to a machine 24 hours a day, which sucked drainage out of my gut. I was too weak to carry it, though it only weighed 5 pounds.

At first, I only got out of bed to use the bathroom, about 10 feet away. For this little trip, someone had to pick up my legs and slowly move them to the floor as I sat up and turned my body to prepare for standing up. Next, they had to help me stand and then walk slowly with me to the bathroom while they carried my machine. I was still thankful I could wipe, a feat I accomplished within an hour of arriving home. The raised toilet seat with arm handles in my bathroom seemed revelatory.

My temperature remained elevated for days, as did my blood pressure. My legs were full of fluid. No one at the hospital had mentioned edema or what to do with my swollen and painful legs, which I already could barely move. Later, after I requested a diuretic medication, the fluid in my legs went away. Being a nurse was helpful. I was fortunate in that.

I was still a prisoner to technology. Day and night, the wound vac machine drained fluid from my gut into a canister attached to the machine on the floor. I worried about it breaking. Sometimes it beeped and I did not know why. A home health nurse came three times a week to change the sponge inside the hole in my abdomen. Sometimes the wound vac company representative met my nurse during her visit. Together they would look at my belly to assess the hole and the machine's role in my healing. Those were early days in the use of wound vac machines. I have since wondered why my attending surgeon chose to use a wound vac to heal my open abdomen instead of more traditional wound care.

Absorbed with the nuances of my new life at home, I had no idea it would take years for me to grasp the full extent of my damages. It was too horrible to imagine I might need another surgery. I did not realize that the removed portion of my small intestine was the location where B12 is absorbed into the body, and therefore I might need B12 injections for the rest of my life. Or that my teeth, damaged from my mouth being open for so long, would require long dental visits and thousands of dollars to redo most of my crowns and fillings. Or that an octave of my singing voice was lost, gone with my breath that no longer allowed me to sustain notes as I had before.

After a life rich with intellectual and analytical discovery, I did not have my usual powers of concentration, though I was not worried about my cognitive function. Surviving each moment while dealing with my physical challenges seemed to be all my brain could handle, and physically surviving was my main agenda. I could not think beyond that.

Reduced to the very basics of my physiological being, I realized I was at the bottom of Maslow's hierarchy of needs. It would be a long time before I got back to self-actualization. For now, I could not wash myself or get dressed without assistance. I could hardly eat, much less cook my food, or even walk to the kitchen. I could not pick up anything or take care of my pets. I could not use my computer because I could not walk up the steps to my office in the loft above my living room. I still could not tolerate television. I was just surviving.

"Uncomfortable time"
–Romeo and Juliet, Act 4, Scene 5

Just 1 month before, except for a cancerous uterus, I was basically a healthy woman. I took no medications. I had no chronic health problems. I could move and carry things without concern. Now, I had 15 to 20 medications to address issues of fever, pain, nausea, constipation, gas, high blood pressure, vitamin deficiency, and more.

My discharge instructions for home care made no mention of my traumatic ordeal. They were written as though I had stayed in the hospital for one uneventful night before going home the next morning. *One hysterectomy*, check. *One night of sleep*, check. *Three tiny abdominal holes healing*, check. *Discharge to home*, check. *See your surgeon at scheduled follow-up appointment*, check.

On the front page was written, "Your thoughts and experiences are important to us. You will soon be receiving a patient satisfaction survey in the mail." I knew the hospital had no interest in knowing what I might have to say. I never got the survey.

Ideal discharge instructions would have included prescriptions for home visits from a shaman to assist in my spiritual respite and renewal, a priest to guide me through meditations of acceptance and forgiveness, a guardian angel to shore up my steadfastness, a Buddhist monk to help me sustain my nonattachment to suffering, Muppets to make me laugh, a massage therapist to realign my energy, a medical sage to give perspective to my calamity, and Shakespeare to poetize my tragedy.

"The thousand natural shocks that flesh is heir to"
–Hamlet, Act 3, Scene 1

My body and psyche had changed. Presumably, the cancer was gone. However, there remained many unintended changes I had to learn to accommodate. The hole in my body and the lost muscle mass were only part of the picture.

Ironically, when I entered the hospital, I felt physically fine. My cancer-ridden uterus did not hurt, producing only occasional drops of blood, though I had begun to identify a deep but dull sensation emanating from that area of my body. Now, I was cancer-free and completely wretched. I had large areas of seminumbness in both legs and thighs and in my right ankle where there seemed to be some nerve damage. I had permanent numbness in my left thumb. My entire abdominal area was numb. I was afraid that if I developed a hernia or another cancer, I would not be able to detect the symptoms. It was weeks before I realized I could hardly sit anywhere, unless upon a cushion, without pain in my buttocks due to nerve damage. I was susceptible to falling out of chairs because of abnormal quick shifts in blood pressure.

"To weep is to make less the depth of grief"
–Henry VI, Part III, Act 2, Scene 1

My heart was broken. I cried every day—tears of anguish, tears of grief. As I began to slowly unravel the trauma of the preceding month, I had very little to go on. Even so, not knowing my recent past and unable to imagine my future, the one thing I knew for certain was that I would be impacted by my physical condition for a long time. It was immediately clear that I was imprisoned in a fortress of useless flesh, physically inert, living in a body so uncooperative that I had only fleeting moments of release through crying. So, when my tears arrived each day, usually in the afternoon, of their own accord, I welcomed the moment, believing they had come to help me cope with surviving this horrific ordeal.

LIFE IN A DAMAGED BODY

*"Sorrow breaks seasons and reposing hours,
makes the night morning, and the noontide night"*
–Richard III, Act 1, Scene 4

Food. I could hardly eat any of it. After weeks of not eating or drinking in the hospital, I had developed dormant taste buds. It was as if my taste buds were deactivated, as though I had never eaten food. I could not tolerate any chemicals, no salt or sugar. I could only eat natural, unprocessed foods. Many of the foods I enjoyed before now tasted awful. One afternoon, a neighbor brought me a plate of homemade chocolate chip cookies, still warm. I could not eat a single morsel, though the friend helping me appreciated the cookies.

Because no one in the hospital explained how common it is for someone who has taken nothing by mouth for weeks to develop intolerance to processed or seasoned foods, I did not realize my taste changes were temporary. I began to mourn the loss of foods I had once enjoyed, fearing I might never be able to eat them again. Eventually, I asked my surgeon about this at an office appointment. He explained that sometimes taste buds *turn over* when they are not used and that anesthesia and certain medications may also contribute to this condition. Later, I did some research and learned that taste dysfunction may be associated with disease and inflammation, a common factor in many diseases (Feng, Huang, & Wang, 2014).

Because I had virtually no appetite, I did not mind not eating. I had gotten used to no food in the hospital. Still, I was strongly encouraged to eat, especially protein—in particular, meat protein—which promoted wound healing. I had not eaten beef or pork for 35 years, so it was excruciatingly difficult to eat the meatloaf or beef stew neighbors offered, though I tried. Whenever I attempted to eat a favorite food, like a sandwich with smoked turkey, Muenster cheese, and mayonnaise, I could not tolerate it.

However challenging it was to eat, I was highly motivated to eat the "right" foods. I needed protein to help heal the huge hole in my stomach. More than anything, I wanted to get well. Through trial and error, I learned I could eat fresh grilled salmon without seasoning, potatoes without butter or sour cream, and fresh fruit and vegetables if they were absolutely plain. I liked to imagine I would become quite thin if I never again ate the overly rich carbohydrate diet I had been accustomed to. I would get a fitness coach and learn how to work out with my mutilated body. I would develop muscle tone to give me shape. I would buy a new wardrobe and eat like a movie star: just salads, grilled chicken, and chardonnay.

If someone in the hospital had told me food would taste odd when I got home, and that it was a temporary aberration, it would have saved me the confusion and concern I felt when I thought I might never eat normally again.

"I . . . am like a drop of water"
–The Comedy of Errors, Act 1, Scene 2

In my final days in the hospital, I had periods of such nausea that even attempting to swallow one sip of water would make me gag. My day nurse constantly reminded me to drink water, but it was almost impossible for me to drink anything. At home, I forgot I was a walking lake, as my college biology professor had described humans, pointing out how much of our bodies is water.

After coming home, I ran a low-grade fever, which sapped what little energy I had, leaving me motionless in bed, just existing. Sometimes, when I stood up after sitting or lying down, I became suddenly dizzy and therefore at risk for toppling over. I slowly figured out that I was experiencing orthostatic (sometimes called postural) hypotension, a condition where blood pressure temporarily drops quickly. Later, I learned my malaise and blood pressure shifts were caused mainly by my not drinking enough liquids, that my temperature and decreased urination were likely caused by dehydration, that I might have felt much better if I had just consumed more water. Something simple can be very significant.

I forgot that I was a lake; that my body was as old as the universe; that the calcium, carbon, and iron in my cells had been created long ago, inside collapsing stars. Had I remembered, it might have given me perspective on both the fragility and eternity of life, regardless of medical mishap. Remembering my ancient origins might have given me a temporary reprieve from the hardships of my body's immediate struggles.

"Sleep seldom visits sorrow;
when it doth, it is a comforter"
—The Tempest, Act 2, Scene 1

For the first time in my life, I had trouble sleeping. When I did sleep, it was not good sleep. However much I needed rest from the daily challenges of my life, sleep was elusive. First of all, I had not slept for a month—the coma did not count. In my final hospital days, following the SICU, I did not sleep. Truly, I did not sleep, as unbelievable as that may sound.

Now home, I could sleep a little, in spite of nightly interruptions, including night sweats, bad dreams, mouth breathing, unexplained fever, discomfort resulting from my inability to reposition my body, pain in my jaw from clenched teeth, overwhelming fear from uncontrollable thoughts, and chronic anxiety about my state of helplessness. Whenever I woke up and realized that miraculously I had been asleep, I found my mouth was open and so dry I could hardly move my tongue to find moisture. Sleep, elusive sleep, was added to my new list of problems—inability to move, weakness, hair loss, anorexia, and insomnia.

It quickly became evident that I could not keep my mouth closed while I slept. No one in the hospital had told me my mouth might stay open for weeks whenever I slept, so it was another problem I had to figure out by myself. I assumed my mouth had been reprogrammed for the open position while it was filled with tubes.

Five years later, I spent $6,000 on dental work to repair the damage to my teeth that had occurred in the hospital, when my open mouth had prevented normal saliva from washing away unhealthy bacteria. Did the SICU staff clean and moisten my teeth and mouth with the correct products often enough?

Another factor affecting my sleep was the wound vac machine. It was supposed to constantly pull drainage out of my body. But what if it broke or stopped working while I was asleep, at 3 a.m., when I would not be able to call anyone to help me? The machine was like a science fiction contraption, ever present on the floor beside my bed, always moving, suctioning my wound, while I passively allowed it.

Then, there was the challenge of my inert body. It made me see what it must feel like to be paralyzed. I could not move my legs in or out of bed. If I needed to pee, I had to summon someone to help me. Early one morning around 2 a.m., a friend sleeping in a nearby bedroom with the door open was unable to hear my calls or my ringing bell. I had to telephone my neighbor next door to ask her to come help me use the bathroom.

What if discharge planners educated patients about some of the problems they might encounter once they got home, especially if their hospital stay was traumatic, lengthy, or involved near-death experiences. Simple knowledge can help people who are otherwise left to worry about things they have no way to understand, when fear looms higher than known realities. I wish someone had talked with me about sleep and pain; changes in body temperature and blood pressure; challenges with balance; alterations in mood; stress-related tightening of body parts (like the jaw); variations in hair, appetite, taste, and such.

Millions of people leave hospitals after physical and medical ordeals and return home with additional problems, like new confusion and suffering, without simple information that might help them experience a better recovery. Although I was a nurse, I did not know about all of this. What if I had been given an informational sheet to take home with this truthful statement, "Please be aware you may develop one or more of these new problems: sleep deprivation, alteration in vital signs such as temperature and blood pressure, temporomandibular joint disorder (TMJ), post-traumatic stress disorder (PTSD), poor appetite, dehydration, fever, edema, loss of hair, dark thoughts, inner terror, loss of hope, increased cynicism about mankind, lack of goodwill and . . ."

"Her hair, her cheek, her gait"
—Troilus and Cressida, Act 1, Scene 1

My hair, my beautiful, once-thick auburn hair, was no more. Within days of arriving home, I could no longer deny it was falling out. By the year's end, I had lost over half of my hair. This was psychologically devastating, especially because no one had told me this might happen.

Why was my hair falling out? Did someone forget to tell me I had chemotherapy or radiation treatments while I was in a coma? Hair loss was just one more thing left out of the needed preparatory education to cover how to be a demoralized, unmoving, broken, homebound patient. I suppose hair loss was a distant runner-up, in terms of significance, when compared to staying alive; maybe that is why it was never discussed. At least I had been told the lymph nodes removed during the hysterectomy surgery had come back "clean," which meant the cancer was completely purged from my body, so I would not need any follow-up treatment.

Hair, I had to figure out on my own. Abandoned patient, heal thyself. After many weeks, I was finally strong enough to research my hair condition and discovered I had *telogen effluvium*—the sudden, unexpected loss of hair caused by severe mental stress or by major illness, surgery, high fever, or severe infection—all of which applied to me.

Hair normally grows in 2- to 5-year cycles. At any given time, most hair is in the growing phase, with less hair in the telogen, or resting, phase. After 2 to 3 months in the telogen phase, resting hairs are pushed out by new hair growth. The severe stress of my hospitalization had caused much of my hair to shift from the growing to the resting phase. People often notice this sudden hair loss 3 to 6 months after a stressful event. Once the stress resolves, shedding usually slows and hair regrows, within 6 to 9 months after the initial loss. My hair was right on schedule.

The first hair stylist I went to said my hair was not long enough to cut. Not until late spring of the following year would I have enough hair for someone to reconcile the longer front and side hair with the new patches of short hair on the back of my head. I once asked my neighbor if the bald spot had any activity. After inspecting the back of my head, she said there was good news and bad news—the little hairs were growing back, but they were coming in gray.

Once I understood why I was losing significant hairs on a daily basis, it was easier to accept. If a clinician had only explained to me about my hair falling out, it would have been easier to deal with my hair loss after I got home.

Caveat: If you tie your hair up before putting on your surgery cap, make sure to tell someone to undo your hair tie if you end up in a coma on a ventilator in the SICU for weeks. Lying on my back, my hair became so gnarled that much of it had to be cut. No one had bothered with my hair for weeks. This I forgave.

FAMILY, FRIENDS, NEIGHBORS, AND COLLEAGUES

"A friend should bear his friend's infirmities"
–Julius Caesar, Act 4, Scene 3

Although I could have gone to a rehabilitation center before going home, I knew I would do better as soon as I got back to my familiar environment. However, someone had to be with me all the time because I could not take care of myself. Having lived alone much of my adult life, I willingly surrendered to my need to have someone help me bathe, eat, and move—and someone to feed the cats, get the mail, answer the telephone, and deal with visitors. It was useful that I had lost all sense of personal privacy while in the hospital.

Not everyone is meant to be a caregiver. The first friend who came to help me was a nurse I had known for years. We had shared many happy hours together, in nature, visiting in each other's homes, sharing delicious meals and interesting talks, and supporting each other in times of need. Although I had explicitly described my situation when I called to ask her to come to be my caretaker for a week, she apparently did not grasp the enormity of my vulnerabilities until she arrived. Almost immediately, I realized she was suffering from being around me, and I began to see a side of her I had never known. I later learned that she was suffering from mental illness and was not well enough to care for me without causing her own suffering.

I soon realized my physical tragedy seemed to make her acutely uncomfortable; it seemed she could not separate herself from what was happening to me. I only needed help to bathe, dress, eat, and move about, which left plenty of time for companionship. I had imagined we would have conversations as we had in the past, covering politics, religion, family, and more. Yet, this undirected time created discomfort and anxiety for her and made the situation unbearable for both of us. It was my first week home from the hospital, and I was experiencing high blood pressure, fever, crying spells, swollen legs, poor sleep, and acute suffering. I was the one who needed help. I could not take care of my own needs, much less hers. Although she had planned to stay for a week, I found someone to relieve her so she could leave sooner.

The next woman who came to help had once been my neighbor in another city. Even though I did not know her well, for some reason I immediately thought to call her for help. She arrived the same day my friend left. It took only moments to adjust to the new bubbly personality in my home. She was talkative, kind, and helpful, and she made me the best scrambled eggs I had ever eaten. She taught me to put whipped cream in my morning coffee, and she read to me. She was like an angel of love and light.

The following week, a woman I had known since grammar school came to help me for a month. She took me to the doctor, washed dishes, ran errands, helped me bathe, and was present for whatever I needed. Whenever she heard me crying, she knew my grief was too deep to give words to, and she gave me space to extinguish the passing storm by myself.

Other people helped me, too. My next-door neighbor was available whenever needed. Colleagues visited, bringing flowers and food. One of them brought me a book about angels. Another one read me *The Velveteen Rabbit*. Some shared the latest news about work. Since I knew it would be at least several months before I could return to work, I relished every tidbit of gossip.

Sisters and other relatives came from time to time, bearing soup, plants, gifts, and well wishes. Longtime friends brought pizza and movies. As though by magic, one friend, a woman I had known as a child and not seen for decades, who lived 3,000 miles away, came to spend part of my birthday week with me. The high school student who helped me with yard work came to visit and talked about becoming an Air Force pilot, which he later accomplished. During Christmas week, a colleague brought me beautiful pearl earrings. Henry, the nurse who helped save my life in the SICU, brought me flowers and good wishes.

CHAPTER 14

TRUTH

"There is no darkness but ignorance"
—Twelfth Night, Act 4, Scene 2

Before I left the hospital, I knew my attending surgeon was culpable for what had happened to me. I was also dependent on him for after-care, so I was carefully polite. Surely he understood my wanting to know how the surgery went wrong, how it had divided my life into two parts: before surgery and after surgery. I did not want to alienate him if there was a chance he might tell me the truth. But I was naïve.

After coming home, I saw him twice a week in his office for a while. Although I had lost trust in him, I never doubted my decision to continue with him. The closer I was to him, the more chance I thought I had to learn the truth. He knew about my surgeries better than anyone, and it made no sense to go to a new surgeon whom I had never seen. I still had no idea how devastating the second (re-pair) surgery was, and how the aspiration had caused the next three surgeries, so my questions focused on the first surgery when my small intestine was injured.

I realize some people might think it odd, or just downright wrong, to continue to see this surgeon, but I forgave him before I came home. I never hated him. How could I be sanguine if I hated him? I needed to keep my mind and heart open, at least until I knew what he had done. In the beginning, he was kindly mute. And I was kindly patient.

I did not see him as a villain. I never thought he intended to hurt
me. Just because I almost died did not mean he did not have expertise. He offered some feedback and assurances, which I appreciated.
To a point, I believed he felt genuine kindness toward me, if for no
other reason than how well we had come to know each other. If my
hysterectomy had been uneventful, I would have gone home the next
day and seen him for one or two check-ups, and then he and I would
have become part of each other's histories.

Although he had failed me, he was a witness to what had happened.
He had been there while I lay unconscious in the operating room.
For the first surgery, then the second one, and the remainder of my
month in the hospital, he was part of my tragedy. He had answers,
but I imagined he could not figure out how to tell me the truth without an apology. He never did apologize, even for my suffering.

Many doctors have trouble apologizing, even though an apology
may lower the risk of a medical malpractice lawsuit. Even when
doctors disclose information, it may be minimal, accompanied by an
incomplete apology. Fear of litigation may be a factor, but so is the
psychological distress of admitting errors. The sad truth is that even
when a doctor is not responsible for something going wrong, and no
matter how much a patient might want to hear it, a doctor may still
find it difficult to say, "I'm sorry" (Mazor et al., 2006).

There is research to show that a doctor's full disclosure about
medical errors produces either a positive effect or no effect on how
patients respond to the medical errors:

> Full disclosure may seem risky to a physician faced with a
> patient who has experienced a medical error, but the results
> presented here suggest that full disclosure is likely to have
> either a positive impact or no impact on patients and family
> members; we found no evidence that full disclosure increases
> the risk of negative consequences for physicians. (Mazor et al.,
> 2006, p. 709)

"Give sorrow words, the grief that does not speak"
–Macbeth, Act 4, Scene 3

I saw my surgeon less and less frequently for more than a year in his office. Each time I found new ways to ask what went wrong. Each time I asked the same question in a different way, changing the wording with each visit, as though the repetition might eventually conjure up the truth. What happened during the surgery to cause my injury? Who applied too much pressure? Were you there? Who else was there?

My attending told me that the surgical approach used to remove lymph nodes from the aorta (staging) had been revised because of my case. He said when my small intestine was moved aside in order to harvest the nodes, it was apparently bruised from the pressure of the instrument. He said what had happened to me was very rare. No one noticed the bruising at the time.

He was careful to talk about instruments, not surgeons, as he described how, after surgery, the two areas of bruising (where each instrument had been clamped) later developed into hematomas (places where blood collects solidly inside the tissue), which then caused blood vessel and muscle to tear away and rupture (perforate) in two places.

Although I understood his description, I knew the graspers did not act independently. I wanted him to connect each grasper with a surgeon. Did the new fellow surgeon hold and manipulate both graspers? Or, did my attending hold and control one of them, while the fellow controlled the second grasper? I suspected the new surgeon had applied too much pressure, and I wanted to know if my attending was right there supervising as well as participating in the procedure. If so, should he have realized the pressure was too great? After

all, the grasper handles were held from outside my body, while inside
a tiny hole, the instrument moved my intestine and then held it in
place. Once, he told me that sometimes a grasper will ratchet down
on its own, maybe with too much pressure, and that this was not
something a surgeon wants to occur. I interpreted that to mean the
surgeon needs to maintain control over the instrument at all times.

One day, he inadvertently began to speak about the nontraumatic
grasper instrument that had been used. Instead of referring to the
grasper, he said the pronoun "we." Before, he had always described
this instrument as though it had its own intelligence, as if it could
manipulate itself without human assistance. Immediately realizing
his mistake, he stopped abruptly. Understanding he could not say,
"*We* applied too much pressure to your small intestine," he slowly
began again. This time, he stated that it was *the grasper's* pressure
that ultimately caused my intestine to break apart. He wanted me
to believe the metal tool was the culprit, not the surgeon holding it. Neither the wise nor the inexperienced surgeon committed
any wrong—even though the surgeon controlled the instrument,
determining how much pressure to use and whether or not to clamp
down on my bowel.

He continued to be elusive, to obfuscate past events with oblique
answers, surely knowing what he was doing, under the guise of his
hurried energy and businesslike manner. He always needed to move
on to his next patient, a valid excuse to avoid answering any more
questions. The more questions he answered, the more likely he
might say something he did not wish to tell.

The wound in my gut did not completely heal until 6 months after I
left the hospital. By then, I was back at work. Occasionally, I saw my
surgeon in the hospital hallway, and he seemed happy to give me a
hug. I welcomed his acknowledgment. Perhaps he felt empathy for
me. In any case, I never forgot that our bond was a direct result of
my trauma at his hands.

"Truth is truth to the end of reckoning"
–Measure for Measure, Act 5, Scene 1

Beware of relying on answers to only the questions you ask. I never asked my attending surgeon about the aspiration because I did not know to ask. It took me a year or more to understand that the botched intubation was a much more serious medical error than my perforated intestine. Truth often lies where you do not know to look.

Doctors are often in a hurry—exhausted, fragmented, or disinterested. They glean the most salient details about your case, and when asked, give back minimal information. There seems to be a pervasive belief that the patient does not need to know much, that immediate essentials will suffice, and that patients should be satisfied to know only what they paternalistically deem is required or important for patients to know. What the doctor understands is always more important than what the patient wants to know, regardless of the concept of patient autonomy. This is paternalism.

My surgeon said very little, virtually ignoring the enormity of my medical debacle. Only when I sought information did he say anything, speaking carefully and minimally. Instead of being honest with me, he chose to protect himself. Early on, I was too sick to realize he had not answered my questions. Only in the car going home, or days later, did I realize he had been evasive, saying something without saying anything, staving off any admission of error. He knew what I yearned to comprehend, what I struggled to have him elucidate. He also knew what he would not disclose.

I believe he hoped I would stop pursuing the truth, that I would give up, that the difficult aftermath of my surgeries might absorb all my attention and squelch any questions still burning inside, that the exacting details of my life in recovery would take precedence over the truth I yearned to know.

When it comes to medical errors, some secrets remain buried. Life moves on. A patient forgets or decides the pursuit of truth is not worth the sacrifice it requires. Regaining physical and emotional well-being may be all-encompassing, leaving little energy for patients to also tackle the Goliath that is medicine's powerful culture. Some may feel that nothing can change the past and that knowing more will not help. At least you are alive. Of course, when you are in a coma, there is nothing you need to know. And justice is just another word, like any other, that you cannot fathom.

"There is some soul of goodness in things evil"
–Henry V, Act 4, Scene 1

Why should my surgeon have placed a higher priority on truth-telling than on his self-interest? He worked in a large medical-industrial complex, an organization whose survival depended upon preserving its own. He was not required to tell me anything the hospital did not want me to know. He was probably forbidden to tell me anything unless the hospital gave him permission.

Before talking with patients and families about unfortunate scenarios, doctors and other staff are usually required to first contact the legal and risk management department, so the hospital and involved parties can get their stories straight and know what to say and what not to say, all for the greater good and best interest of the hospital's liability and financial interests. There is an emphasis on taking great care and thought before sharing potentially detrimental information. This culture of fear makes it seem as if the patient's own health and safety falls at the bottom of the priority list. It can make a hospital seem less like a place of healing and more like an incubator of secrets.

I blamed the hospital system as much, if not more, as my surgeon for not telling me the truth. My surgeon, along with the hospital and my healthcare insurance company, was on one side of the scale of justice, with me on the other side. If passion were going to tip the balance, it would need to be my passion.

Doctors generally must adhere to hospital policies that affect patient care. My surgeon was a cog in the great organizational wheel. As A. K. Edwin indicates in his 2009 journal article about the nondisclosure of medical errors:

> Although most doctors believe that errors should be disclosed to patients when they occur, in reality, most doctors and institutions do not disclose such mishaps to patients and their families. Rather, they engage in extensive cover ups under the guise of protecting the doctor-patient relationship and not causing harm to patients. . . . By not disclosing a medical error, the doctor conspicuously places his own interests above that of the patient to the detriment of the patient, thereby violating a patient-centered ethic. Moral courage is therefore needed if doctors are to do the right thing when medical errors occur. This moral courage can be facilitated by institutions having policies and guidelines on disclosure of errors in place, training doctors and other hospital staff on how to disclose medical errors and providing emotional support for doctors who make mistakes in their efforts to treat patients and save lives. (p. 34)

Because of my experiences with the institutional wall of resistance, I was interested and delighted to learn that some hospital systems do better. For example, in 2001–2002, the University of Michigan Health System (UMHS) began to promote patient safety through the principles of honesty, transparency, and accountability, by changing its approach to risk management through an early disclosure and offer (D&O) program (Boothman, Imhoff, & Campbell, 2012). This program was:

> Informed by two central observations: (1) honesty is indispensable for safety improvement, and (2) a short-term focus on financial risk impedes long-term improvement. The tenets of the D&O system include compensating patients quickly and

fairly when inappropriate medical care causes injury, communicating openly with patients about error(s), supporting staff vigorously when appropriate care has been provided, and reducing future injuries and claims through application of knowledge garnered through the discovery process. (Boothman & Hoyler, 2013, p. 21)

Other hospitals would do well to study what UMHS has accomplished in the last decade. Its "D&O model has successfully resulted in fewer claims, fewer lawsuits, and lower liability costs," (Boothman & Hoyler, 2013, p. 23), while making every effort to put patients and their safety first and also "serving and protecting physicians, providers, and health system" (p. 25).

How very different my story might have turned out if only the hospital where I stayed for a month had operated like the University of Michigan Health System.

LIVING IN FEAR

"The best safety lies in fear"
—Hamlet, Act 1, Scene 3

Fear lives in the future, in the dark unknown. At times, I would dive straight into fear, fascinated by the unbelievable drama unfolding in my life. Mostly, I took each moment as it came, both in the hospital and after I got home. I was a warrior. I had many things to fear, but I could be fearful and fearless at the same time.

I was afraid of my body. I tried not to think of it as my enemy, because I could not get away from it. But I was constantly afraid of moving incorrectly, especially since I could not feel certain areas of my body, including my gut. I worried about picking up something too heavy and then needing hernia surgery, or falling and breaking something and needing orthopedic surgery. I worried about having cancer again, or getting some new terrible disease. Just because I had survived thus far did not mean I was immune to further bad luck. I began to live my life devoid of spontaneous movement.

Years earlier, like many young women, I struggled to embrace my physical self. I remember once, in my early 20s, holding up a mirror to see my naked backside in the closet mirror. I looked at my buttocks and the curve of my back in disbelief, as though I was staring at a stranger's body. Looking at my naked self that day, I pledged to unify my consciousness and form.

From that day, I began to see I had a lovely body, voluptuous and smooth-skinned. After the demise of an early marriage, I claimed my sexual power. Men desired me, and I felt I could be with whomever I chose. I made love for pure pleasure.

Before my surgery and subsequent deterioration, I could run and dance, joyful in the exhilaration of using my body without thinking about it, no holding back. My legs were strong enough to carry me wherever I wanted to go, across the earth forever. I remember walking on the beach, bare feet on warm sand, feeling the power and strength of the ocean while firmly grounded on the shifting sand with every step. Now, I could not take any step for granted.

I came home from the hospital feeling like spoiled goods: damaged, scarred, and impaired. I worried about nerve-damaged places in my legs, knowing I could not sit on hard surfaces because of the pain. My blood pressure continued to cause me to fall unpredictably. After not using my legs for a month, they were very weak. My core, the center of my body, had been ruined. I had no belly button. I struggled with my body image and worried that a man might never feel desire toward me again, though I worked hard to let that fear go. I had to wiggle sideways like an earthworm to get out of a prone position. I could not rise up from sitting without pushing off from the chair with my arms. Always, I had to think about my insides, since much of my abdominal region was still numb.

What scared me even more was the degree to which my lungs had been injured in the hospital. The aspiration that occurred during my emergent intubation caused me to lose part of my air-exchange function. Sometimes I ruminated about the possibility of developing lung cancer and chronic obstructive lung disease. What if new disease was already plotting to take over my tissue? I had grown up in a home with two smoking parents and later smoked myself. Thankfully I had stopped long ago, but would that have been soon enough?

I still worried about my hysterectomy, the initial surgery. What if the surgeons had caused the cancer to spread beyond my uterus? The harvested lymph nodes had tested negative—no cancer. But what if the surgeons had also done this part of my surgery incorrectly? What if they had seeded my insides with cancer cells? If I lived with a ticking time bomb inside me, how and when would I know?

After meeting with my attorney a few days after I came home from the hospital, she and I, and eventually others, spent many hours over the next 2 years scrutinizing my medical records and talking with experts who gave feedback to us about relevant portions, especially the anesthesiology part of my second surgery. It took me a year or more to realize that my aspiration was by far the riskiest event I suffered, even though without the initial bowel perforation, I would not have needed that repair surgery or the surgeries that came after that.

Along with my ongoing research while writing this book, I learned something important I had never realized: that preventable hospital medical errors are a major leading cause of death in this country. In a 2013 study, John James explores his estimate that at least 440,000 hospital patients each year suffer some type of preventable harm that contributes to their death.

On July 17, 2014, at a U.S. Senate Subcommittee hearing on Primary Health and Aging, there was testimony that medical errors are the third leading cause of death in the United States. Senator Bernie Sanders (D-Vermont) said that "medical harm is a major cause of suffering, disability, and death—as well as a huge financial cost to our nation" (U.S. Senate, 2014). Joanne Disch, PhD, RN, in her statement to the committee, noted that it was not just daily deaths that should be a huge cause for alarm, but the 10,000 serious complications cases that result from medical errors occurring daily.

In addition to my ongoing concerns about my body, I worried about dying before I achieved my life's purpose, whatever that might be. Most of all, I worried about needing more surgery, which is exactly what happened 14 months later.

"What's to come is still unsure"
—*Twelfth Night,* Act 2, Scene 3

From time to time, my surgeon had quietly mentioned I would likely need repair surgery to put my abdominal cavity back together. Knowing how abhorrent the idea of more surgery was for me, he gently explained that the slowly forming, paper-thin scar tissue over the hole in my abdomen, which had taken 6 months to form, would not safely protect what lay beneath. It took me almost a year to accept that to avoid surgery would put myself at greater risk than to have it; my abdominal muscles were still retracted to each side of my belly, making me vulnerable to injury.

A year and several months after I left the hospital, swearing I would never have surgery again, I chose a different doctor and a different hospital and prepared to go under the knife. The surgeon I selected came highly recommended, especially by other surgeons and medical professionals. He had the reputation of being one of the best. I checked him out with my malpractice attorney, whose firm had the goods on every physician in the city and county. I asked my medical friends and colleagues about him. If they knew him, they had only high praise. Before our first meeting, I carefully prepared for him a summary so he would know my history:

Summary of Prior Surgeries:

Day 1—Dx Uterine Cancer

Day 16—Laparoscopic removal of uterus, during which the surgeons failed to notice my small intestine (distal ileum) had been injured (bruised) in two places.

Day 18—CT scan with contrast showed perforation in two bruised areas of small intestine.

Day 18—10 cm section of small intestine (between two hematoma/perforated areas) removed and intestine stapled together; problems with intubation caused aspiration, which resulted in chemical burns to lungs, pneumonia, ARDS, sepsis. Required three subsequent surgeries. I was maintained in a coma and ventilated in the Surgical ICU for 18 days.

Day 25 and Day 27—Two surgeries to wash out infection in pelvic and abdominal areas.

Day 30—Fifth surgery to close abdomen; the infection had eroded tissue and fascia; muscles left in retracted position on each side of abdomen; bioderm placed (to prevent future herniation); wound vac left in place over an approximately 9 X 15 cm area.

Day 36—Left the SICU.

Day 44—Discharged home from hospital.

Day 45 to Day 113—Home health RN care.

Day 106—Wound vac out, wound still open, now with tunnel (3–4 cm at top of wound/scar area); wound care continues. [Tunneling occurs when a channel forms from the wound into and through subcutaneous tissue, usually caused by infection.]

Day 218—Wound finally closes and wound care stops.

After he read it, we began to talk, as he maintained steady eye contact with me. At one point, I said, *You seem to be paying attention to me!* He replied that he was certainly trying to listen. I decided on this basis alone that he was no ordinary surgeon.

He explained that my last surgery was an intermediary (temporary) surgery. Whoever performed it was correct not to put permanent mesh into my body, given the raging infection I had suffered, since permanent mesh contains material that poses a higher risk of infection. He said it was good I had waited the past year before having surgery, but now it was time to put my abdominal muscles back in their proper place and cover my abdominal organs with skin. Otherwise, the paper-thin scar tissue would ultimately fail to keep my organs safe. The scar tissue, plus the temporary covering placed inside me a year before, had evolved to take on the characteristics of whatever surrounded it, as though it had become muscle. Yet, it was not protective enough for me to live that way for the rest of my life. I needed surgery.

He was confident he could perform the complicated surgery and seemed excited by the challenges it presented. After having another CT of my abdomen, surgery was set for early December. The surgery would take about 2 hours, followed by a 5- to 7-day hospital stay, and then a 6-week recovery. He said I might have 20 to 30 more years of life and should enjoy as high a quality of life as possible, adding that I would carry a 10% chance of needing a future repair surgery, because that was the nature of things. At worst, he would not be able to reposition the muscles back together, meaning, he would not be able to make me whole again.

"True hope is swift, and flies with swallow's wings"
–Richard III, Act 5, Scene 2

Hope is buying new furniture before your Pap smear result comes back. Hope is looking forward to a future, to a meaningful life.

For me to choose to lie unconscious in sterile wrapping, while a doctor cut into me, I needed hope. And faith. Faith that I had chosen an excellent and honest surgeon, faith that he would protect me, that my pain and suffering would be worth enduring so I could have a stronger body and live longer. I made him promise me there would be no medical students or new doctors or observers in the operating room during my surgery. He assured me that only he and his surgical team would be present to perform the operation. I believed him because I trusted him.

I wrote this letter the day before surgery, hoping it would cover any tragic scenario that might again befall me:

I hope all goes well with my surgery tomorrow and that I come home in a timely fashion and recover to where my body works better than it did before the surgery. I want to return to work and finish my book.

However, if something happens during my hospitalization that might require invasive surgery, like a coronary bypass surgery, I do not want that. I would rather die than go through anything additional to what I am dealing with.

I do not want heart surgery.

I do not want brain surgery.

I am okay with dying.

This debacle I have been through for more than a year is enough. Tomorrow is supposed to be a repair of the prior damage to my body, inasmuch as it can be repaired. Yet, my body will never be as it was. And there may be complications down the road, secondary to last year and tomorrow's repair surgery.

I can make my own decisions about what I want if I am conscious. But if I am unable to know what is happening, please remember my wishes. There are too many "what ifs," and I could not name them all if I tried.

I do not want to regain consciousness and be worse off than I was before, like if I have a stroke or heart attack during the surgery and end up paralyzed or brain dead. I cannot go through another major recovery period, especially if it is worse than what I have already experienced. I would rather my life end and cut my losses than go through another medical tragedy.

"Such men are dangerous"
–*Julius Caesar,* Act 1, Scene 2

Although I had faith in my new surgeon to protect me while I was unconscious, I knew there would be other impediments. But I did not anticipate they would occur prior to the next surgery.

At my pre-op appointment, I began to explain to the anesthesiologist that I did not want any student or new doctor involved with my surgery and would so initial on the consent form. He became visibly upset and demanded to know why. I explained how a student had incorrectly intubated me the year before, causing me to aspirate, which set off a cascade of traumatic consequences. Visibly angry, he lectured me, talking to me like I was an idiot who did not know what I was talking about. He arrogantly insisted that:

- People may believe something went wrong but they are just ignorant and do not really understand the facts.

- Nurse anesthetists are excellent—he should know—he trains them.

- There may have been a physical anomaly or some other explanation for what happened to me, but he doubted the intubation was done incorrectly.

- Patients are not allowed to make any exceptions or alterations or requests related to the consent form for surgery, and this is ironclad. And if I did, I would have to go somewhere else for my surgery. *(Wrong)*

I was not going to argue with him or be deterred from my request. I said I felt a lot of tension between us and left it at that. Then, the pre-op nurse, whom I had asked to contact the hospital's risk management department about my request, returned to the cubicle to tell me (and the anesthesiologist) that, yes, a patient does have the right to cross out certain items, with initials, and to add additional information, before signing the consent form. He looked incredulous and said nothing.

I spent the weekend before surgery writing a letter to the anesthesiologist's supervisor, describing his rude, inappropriate, and unprofessional treatment toward me. His ego-bound need to prove me wrong so he could be right was unnecessary. His rebuke had sapped my energy and made an already scary situation even worse. A week later, after I came home from the hospital, the supervisor called to apologize, saying the matter would be dealt with.

I have since learned that anesthesia-related errors can be more dangerous than surgical errors, because even a small error by the anesthesiologist can cause permanent injury, brain damage, or death. Common anesthesiology errors include giving the patient too much anesthesia, failing to properly monitor vital signs, or improperly intubating the patient. A 2014 study (Ranum, Ma, Shapiro, Chang, & Urman) found that the most frequent injuries related to anesthesia involved damage to teeth, patient death, nerve damage, organ damage, pain, and cardiopulmonary arrest.

"What wrong else may be imagined"
–"The Rape of Lucrece"

I woke up after the repair surgery in a psychedelic morphine sky of diamonds, dazzled by rainbow halos, all while various staff cared for my tubes. Five days later, I went home to experience the kind of pain that makes you cry out at merely the thought of moving. Because I remembered no pain during my month in the hospital the previous year, except for one long bout of gas pain toward the end, this kind of extreme pain was new to me. With a fresh, foot-long cut from my pubic bone to the top of my abdominal cavity, I was rent asunder by pain I had never before consciously experienced, pain so acute I could not contain my mournful shrieks, pain beyond the reach of opioids.

Severe pain torments; it sends you into the highest realms of living hell, each moment seems eternal, the agony obscures all memory. Horrific pain can transform you into a creature debilitated and consumed by a wretched force so powerful it completely obliterates who you used to be. You are not dead, though you might wish it so. Inside physical suffering of such magnitude, there is no space for anything else, no past, no future, no time, no realm of hope or prayer. There is only primal terror that the pain will never stop, terror that takes hold and does not let go until it has run its course.

Home from the hospital, with no IV morphine or tubes or nursing staff to help me with bodily functions, I began to experience literally gut-wrenching pain whenever I had to move my body up or down. Sometimes it took me half an hour to gather enough courage to push my body upright to a sitting position, from which I could eventually stand and leave the bed. The pain was so great I could not move without crying out. My narcotic pain medicine was minimally effective.

To give meaning to my physical suffering, I used Tonglen, a Tibetan Buddhist breathing meditation for connecting with the suffering of others. As I breathed in, I visualized taking in the suffering of all people who experience horrific physical pain. As I breathed out, I sent prayers of comfort and peace to those in the agony of pain. My silent meditation for me was: *Now I finally know this kind of pain, this agony that ends who I am in this moment; may my visceral experience help me better empathize with others and be a better teacher and nurse.*

During the complicated surgery, my entire abdomen had been vertically split open. Tissue was cut away or moved. Muscles were rearranged and overlaid with a mesh screen to protect my intestines while my abdomen healed. As my surgeon manipulated, cut, separated, and rearranged my intestines and organs to put my abdomen back together, pain receptors were activated, producing the acute pain I felt when I came home without a morphine pump to help me. He also created for me a new navel, which I had not thought to request.

He found excessive scar tissue (adhesions) from my previous five surgeries. Meticulously, he had to cut through scar tissue to carefully separate sections of my bowel that were stuck together *(lysis of adhesion)*. He removed parts of the bowel that were too damaged to be repaired. Unexpectedly, he had to cut away another 10 cm in the same area where my small intestine had been repaired the first time. Then he reconnected *(anastomosed)* the new ends back together. The surgery took 4 hours instead of the 2 hours he had estimated, which meant I was at increased risk for infection. Instead of using the polyurethane mesh screen, as originally planned, he used donor tissue, which he said was less likely to cause problems with post-op infection.

I never imagined I would wake up after surgery with a new affliction, a seroma—a pocket of clear serous fluid. This (extracellular) fluid, found outside the tissue cells inside various body cavities, bathes and surrounds the cells. When surgery causes small blood vessels to rupture, this fluid builds up. Typically, people who have gastrointestinal surgery have drains inserted to collect fluid buildup inside the abdominal cavity.

Prior to surgery, my surgeon had asked my permission to use a wound vac machine to collect this fluid, instead of surgically implanting drains as was customarily done. Although he said he had never used a wound vac for this kind of extensive abdominal surgery, he thought it might significantly lower my risk for infection, since, unlike internal drains, the machine would cause continuous drainage of this fluid.

Unfortunately, the wound vac did not work, at all. My surgeon and I were disappointed that no fluid was removed by the machine. By the second day after surgery, he had removed the wound vac; however, he could not take me back to surgery to insert drains. He said he did not understand why the wound vac did not work, but that the serous fluid would eventually disperse within my body.

The fluid inside my gut caused my belly to bulge out like a giant fluid-filled tumor, swinging below my waist when I walked. It was like a huge watermelon under my skin, an appendage so heavy I had to wrap it with an abdominal binder and then hold my abdomen with both hands in order to move. Later, I regretted giving my permission to use the wound vac.

I went home with a large elastic wrap, which was used to hold my swollen abdomen whenever I was upright. But after 3 days at home, I went to my surgeon's office, crying before I began to talk. He inserted a big syringe into my belly and drained several quarts of fluid into a large container. He explained that removing the fluid with a syringe increased my risks for infection, but he saw no other choice. I had to go back two more times for this procedure. The seroma was bulky and uncomfortable and became the most difficult aspect of my recovery.

After several weeks, the seroma finally went away, and the physical pain from my reorganized abdominal area subsided. Not once did I doubt that my surgeon had done his very best to help me. I continued to have faith in him. I trusted him to tell me the truth, no matter what. Throughout this time of healing, we made decisions together. I saw him about a dozen times before my body stabilized.

The events of the past year and a half continued to haunt me and filled me with fear of what might come. I doubted I would ever have enough fortitude to enter a hospital again. Death might be better than undergoing another surgery. While I did not actively think of suicide, knowing death would end my misery gave me some comfort.

I was no longer the woman I used to be, not just because my body was different but because my mind and heart had changed. My trust in the world had further diminished, while my vigilant attention to detail had strengthened. Feeling betrayed by doctors and a medical system that seemed stacked against patients, I felt a new hardened place in my spirit.

Would I become a better person or a more tragic figure? Would my wounding make me morally stronger, or would my tragic circumstances cause my gradual disintegration?

FACING DEATH AGAIN

"Life's but a walking shadow"
—Macbeth, Act 5, Scene 5

A year after my painful repair surgery, I was once again facing a potential death scenario. I began to see my future disappearing as thoughts and feelings about dying flooded back into me. This unfathomable turn of events began when I looked in the mirror one day and noticed an odd curvature along my spine, between my neck and back. I called my primary doctor, who had not noticed the anomaly in a recent annual physical exam. She arranged for me to get a thoracic spine X-ray.

I had the X-ray the following week. Before my doctor called, I received my copy of the radiology report in the mail. I quickly read the radiologist's foreboding words of concern over something called *superior mediastinal prominence*, which might indicate that I had a disease of the lymph nodes *(lymphadenopathy)*. In other words, my pulmonary veins and arteries—as well as my cardiac veins and aorta (great vessels) and my trachea and esophagus—might be misplaced due to a malignancy or an autoimmune disease. Something might be wrong deep inside my chest cavity, around my heart, between my lungs. It was not good.

Immediately, I went online to research these potential conditions. My fears quickly grew. According to what I read, there was a real possibility that I might have lung cancer, acute lymphocytic leukemia, or lymphoma. Once again, just as I did 3 years ago when I first learned I had cancer, I went to bed, filled with existential despair.

I needed a CT scan of my chest, which was scheduled for the following week. As I awaited the specifics of my potential new death sentence, hours seemed like days. Once again, I was a tragic figure in my own life and contemplating death.

To cope, I tried to stay in the moment, where attention to detail became a saving grace. I did normal things. I talked on the phone, answered emails, ran errands, watched television, read the newspaper, and walked my dog. I had been on this path before. Thankfully, I knew how to be present in my body, to be aware of thoughts without believing them. Living in the present moment became my refuge, just like it had 2 years earlier, while I was conscious in the hospital.

I took comfort in knowing I had prepared (as much as possible) for my good death. I maintained current advance directives—legal documents that spell out the terms of how I want to die and who will speak for me if I am unable to communicate. Like many people who create these directives, I had a living will stating I wanted to die a natural death and a healthcare power of attorney naming people to be my voice if I became unable to speak for myself. Perhaps most importantly, I did not have any regrets, having long ago granted absolution for everyone and everything.

"That we shall die we know,
tis but the time
and drawing days out,
that men stand upon"
–Julius Caesar, Act 3, Scene 1

After the CT scan, I called the radiologist who had interpreted the results. I was amazed to learn that, though we had never met, she remembered me, or at least she remembered my lungs. She was the radiologist on call the day of my repair surgery the year before and still remembered looking at the images of my lungs and body during that surgery.

Happily, she informed me that I had no shifted mediastinum; that the radiology technician who performed the thoracic spinal X-ray had probably positioned me incorrectly, thus causing a shadow that appeared to be a suspicious mass. She knew how damaged my lungs had once been, and, unbelievably, she told me, "Your lungs are gorgeous!" It was almost worth going through a major health scare due to a technician's faulty work just to hear her say this.

Not really; it was not worth it.

"Merely players"
–As You Like It, Act 2, Scene 7

Long before I got cancer, I learned that suffering is universal. To suffer is to be human. To open and feel this suffering is to have compassion for one's self, and thereby for others. Suffering connects each of us to all of humanity; it is the gateway to the interconnectedness of all things.

Throughout the last 3 years of medical drama and fear, I maintained a sense of compassion for my suffering and for myself, as well as for those who cared for me. Many years earlier, I had been greatly influenced by a book first published in 1978 titled *The Road Less Traveled*, in which M. Scott Peck teaches that only when we accept that life is difficult for everyone can we learn to deeply feel our personal anguish and reach a higher truth.

Before I got cancer, I had always been a seeker of truth, learning to see my life as a precious mystery in good and bad times, understanding that my life was more than a series of problems to be solved. My life was my spiritual journey. Cancer, hospital, surgery, coma—these were new problems I learned to transcend.

THE POWER OF SUFFERING

"To fear the worst, oft cures the worse"
–Troilus and Cressida, Act 3, Scene 2

My childhood prepared me for surgery gone wrong. As a baby, I had no intellectual capacity to understand why my father angrily spanked my legs to get me to stop crying. I was born to young parents with personal demons, and I lived out an abusive childhood. Because of the violence, I learned to go deep inside myself. I would come back out when the coast was clear, usually late at night. I would lie in my bed listening to the radio, while my sisters and parents slept upstairs. I created a fantasy world to escape my invisible prison.

Adolescence provided me with different ways to escape my family demons by leaving home. I developed sexual lust at a young age, though I did not understand or know what to do with it. In high school I spent the night at my girlfriends' homes, and we sneaked out to parties with university students. I drank vodka and apple juice and stayed up all night. My parents never knew. I also learned how to play guitar and began performing as a folk singer in a local coffee house. Away from home, I felt free.

As a young woman, I began to leave behind my depressed childhood, without realizing I had been depressed. I let go of a lifetime of being unloved and mistreated, without realizing I was forgiving. I began to look at people when I talked with them. I stopped using "I'm sorry" to begin or end sentences. Somehow, my backlog of heartbreak guided me toward the light. I became a spiritual athlete. I learned how to love my self, without realizing I was opening the door to loving others, especially the people who had damaged me. At times, the boundaries between me and everything else dissolved, leaving me without ego, though I had no words to describe this phenomenon.

Suffering was my spiritual teacher, always training me to be resilient. And curious.

Behind my suffering was an insatiable desire to understand myself and my life, to know why, to see beyond my hardships. As each decade unfolded, I wanted to know what would happen next on my journey. As I anticipated my cancer surgery, I wondered how I would fare emotionally. Would I deepen spiritually? Then, after almost dying, I wondered how much time I had left and if I would be able to recreate my good life.

"Pain pays the income of each precious thing."
−"The Rape of Lucrece"

Suffering is often silent and invisible, unmarked by the tears or cries of physical pain. Sometimes suffering resides so deep within us that it cannot be seen or understood by those on the outside.

Although I had experienced the rhythms of sorrow that move through all of us, I was unprepared for the terror I felt when I woke up that day in the SICU with no memory, imprisoned in a body that did not work. I did not know where I was. I did not know who I was. I could not even comprehend I was suffering. My fear and dread overwhelmed me.

Even if I could have spoken during those first moments after I was taken off the ventilator, and drugs were withdrawn, and consciousness seeped back into my brain cells, my horror would have been too big for words as "I" no longer existed. Unable to leave the moment, and without the ability to self-reflect, I had no concept of anything.

There was no "me" to experience despair. Had I been able to construct thoughts, they would have been, *I am in very bad trouble; I do not know the details.*

I never forgot the way I felt that day in the SICU. Ten months later, as I stood beside my mother's hospital bed, in my childhood bedroom, in the house where my mother had lived for more than 50 years, I felt a powerful connection with how I imagined she might be feeling. She was dying from one of her illnesses, possibly the metastatic breast cancer or the dementia. She was on oxygen and had a catheter. She had been with hospice for a year. Now, she was close to death. She had not spoken more than a few words for weeks. Her eyes stayed mostly closed, which I later realized was to minimize the stimulation of her environment.

Looking at her, in silence, I tried to imagine her suffering, what it felt like to have no words to frame what was happening to her, no speech to connect with her daughters. Did she know she had passed the point of no return? That it was too late now to talk of her plight with us, that her oblivion was too advanced?

Before, when she might have shared her fear and depression over what she suspected was changing her brain, she refused to do so, no matter how we tried to acknowledge her angst about what was occurring. As we watched her disappear, we soothed her brow and comforted and witnessed her, until her brain literally took her away before her body died.

"The quality of mercy is not strained.
It droppeth as the gentle rain from heaven
upon the place beneath. It is twice blessed:
It blesseth him that gives and him that takes."
–*The Merchant of Venice*, Act 4, Scene 1

Because I forgave my mother decades before she died, I was able to spend time with her. Eventually, I forgave the surgeons who hurt me, so I could move on with my life.

I understood the history of training a doctor to see the patient's body and mind as separate, lest medical objectivity be compromised. Although medical education continues to evolve, many practicing doctors were not trained to understand the mind-body connection. Today, many medical students are still taught to objectify the patient, to believe emotional involvement will distort their medical expertise. Beyond the immediacy of physical pain and limitation, physicians often fail to recognize the invisible yet powerful dimensions of patient suffering: loneliness, hopelessness, and powerlessness.

If it is possible for physicians to stop viewing their patients as consumers of services and instead see them as human beings who need care, how can it be done? True compassion replaces "niceness" when physicians understand that suffering is about more than a broken body, that it encompasses a person's mind and spirit, hopes and dreams, sense of control, and fears about what is to come. We need our caregivers to offer compassion, not superficially wrapped pleasantries. Patients struggle to create meaning around what is happening to them, and they need to share humanity with the people rendering care.

Suffering is not just the domain of patients. It also affects the physicians and nurses who care for patients. Seeing suffering causes suffering, but often suffering is invisible. If a nurse or doctor believes suffering does not exist beyond physical pain, then they have no responsibility beyond the medication and physical tasks required to address it. When healthcare providers are educated and trained to see their patients holistically, they learn to be fully engaged and are able to give better care. They also derive energy from such encounters.

Eric Cassell (1991), who wrote *The Nature of Suffering and the Goals of Medicine*, explains that when we open our hearts, we see our patients as individuals with needs beyond medical science, not as objectified customers. Working with patients through heart-centered care requires no extra energy or time. Seeing the suffering around us is not a function of what we do but of who we are. Only through seeing suffering can we begin to ameliorate it. Cassell writes:

> Now comes the hard part: learning to be simply open in the presence of the patient, as though there were a door to the inside of you—to your heart or soul, call it what you will—and you consciously opened it so the patient would flow into you. (1999, p. 534)

Being nice may suffice in a checkout line at the grocery store. We do not need to feel a sense of humanity with the cashier who prices our vegetables. However, when our health or life is at stake, while we lie in the foreign land of a hospital as our former life dissolves with no new future yet in focus; when our personal identity is temporarily destroyed, and we struggle to understand the enormity of what we are losing—in these moments, a superficial pleasantry may seem worthless, even insulting.

CHAPTER 18

THE SUFFERING OF OTHERS

"Oh, I have suffered with those that I saw suffer"
—The Tempest, Act 1, Scene 2

Nurses and doctors, as well as nursing and medical students, suffer moral distress when they lack the ethical framework to help their patients deal with difficult decisions and life-threatening situations. According to Whitehead et al. (2015), regardless of healthcare profession, moral distress is a common experience for clinicians.

Nurses and doctors suffer moral distress when they lack the training and insight to utilize ethical frameworks for good patient care and decision-making. Epstein and Delgado (2010) report that:

> Moral distress occurs when one knows the ethically correct action to take but feels powerless to take that action. Research on moral distress among nurses has identified that the sources of moral distress are many and varied and that the experience of moral distress leads some nurses to leave their jobs, or the profession altogether. (p. 1)

Having taught a course every year on ethical issues in nursing practice, I am well aware of how crucial ethics training is for nursing students, especially for those who end up working in medical and surgical intensive care units, where life and death struggles are common. At the end of the course, my students frequently commented that they could not imagine entering the professional realm of nursing without at least some knowledge of how to formulate the ethically right course of action in the kinds of situations they knew they would encounter.

In nursing education, medical ethics is seldom required and some-times not even offered, perhaps due to the shortage of faculty who know how to teach this curriculum. As Jeanette Der Bedrosian reported in 2015, "There's a nationwide shortage of nursing faculty, and only a small percentage of those instructors have been educated in ethics" (p. 27). The report went on to say that many who do lead ethics courses have no formal background.

Throughout my career, I have listened to many nurses describe situations in which they were not allowed to pursue the ethically right course of action for their patients, or when they felt inadequate to help their patients in difficult circumstances. One nurse told me about an evening when she was not allowed to give her patient, a young woman, the ordered pain medication because the parents did not want their daughter to have it. The nurse was still upset that her patient suffered because of physical pain that could have been mitigated.

In class as well as in clinical settings, nurses have told me stories about being forbidden to share information with an older adult patient because a family member did not want the patient to know. This sometimes happened in spite of the patient's former wishes and advance directives.

I have heard many stories from nurses who knew doctors, especially new ones, were not doing what was best for the patient, either from being in a hurry or from not realizing the full extent of what was needed. Nurses have often told me how they feared speaking up, especially in a culture where virtually everyone values doctors more than nurses. They have shared with me their suffering over knowing the patient was not getting the right care, and they felt helpless to intervene.

In these situations, the nurses might have known other ways to ad-vocate for their patients, if they: (1) had education in nursing school and training at work about the ethical issues they might encounter, and how to understand and apply concepts of autonomy, justice, beneficence, nonmaleficence, truth-telling, and respect, all of which are essential for best nursing practice; and (2) had been taught and trained together with medical students to understand each other's professional roles and to learn how best to collaborate for the patient's highest good.

In my last semester of nursing school, I took care of a beautiful young doctor who was dying. She had worked as a physician with a poor, rural population until she got sick with cancer. After treatment, she returned to her patients only to have the cancer return with a vengeance. I was in her room about to expose her buttock for an injection when in walked a doctor with a flock of medical trainees trailing behind to see the next specimen. They did not knock or ask permission to enter the room. In a second, without thinking, I heard myself say, "Please leave; I am getting ready to give my patient an injection." The medical herd turned around without comment and left the room. Thinking nothing of this, I commenced to care for my patient.

Only later in my career did I realize how unusual it was for a (female) nursing student to speak up for her patient against a group of doctors and medical students. Why did I do it? Did I feel courageous that day? I do not remember taking any time to get up my nerve. My comment to the doctors was spontaneous and immediate. I was not aware of feeling *ethical*. Was my age a factor in speaking up? After all, I was older than most of my classmates because I came to nursing school after earning two college degrees. Was my background a factor? Perhaps yes. I grew up in a home where principles of justice were often woven into dinner conversations. Or maybe it was because I had taken seriously the caveat in nursing school—that a nurse's foremost duty is to protect her patient, to be both advocate and caregiver.

"They breathe truth that breathe their words in pain"
–Richard II, Act 2, Scene 1

I know suffering as a patient, nestled inside singularity, suspended between who I was and who I may become: *I am here. Can you see me? Do you know me? Can you honor me? Am I going to die? If I recover, how will my life change? Am I doomed to misery for the rest of my life?*

I know suffering as a nurse. Behind my patients' faces, I can see what they cannot speak.

As a teacher, I know the suffering of my students. I see them struggle to keep from activating their personal wounds while they interact with mentally ill patients, before they have figured out there is little difference between them and their patients: *I am becoming someone else. I am no longer who I was. Will opening my heart to a patient diminish me in some way?*

I understand suffering of people imprisoned in their bodies, disconnected from the external, as they drown in despair, delirium, amnesia, or silence: *I am not who you see; I am not where you see me; I am someone else. Please do not forsake me.*

I see suffering from loss of self, from powerlessness, from a diminishing which empties the human vessel of even the possibility for redemption or joy: *I live on the streets. Nobody truly knows me. I make no difference to myself or to the world. If I die no one will notice.*

Suffering is not confined to bodies; it lives inside the psyche, beyond temporal condition, beyond words.

Suffering is invisible, isolating, separating. When I share my humanity with you, I witness and connect with your experience. *As I see me, I see you. As I see you, I am you.*

If I view you as an object to manipulate, or a body to objectify, I rob us both of humanity. *We are the same person.*

If my heart is open, if I can see myself, I will also see you, even if you cannot see me, even if you are powerless, defeated, hidden, or lost. *We are the same person.* If you cannot speak, if you do not have the words, I will be your voice. *We are the same person.*

Each morning as light seeps onto my bed and brightness pulls my sleeping body out of dreams into a new day, I feel my breath and check my beating heart as the human story reactivates inside my consciousness. I ask myself, how does it matter that I am alive?

THE PERSON INSIDE THE PATIENT

*"We know what we are,
but know not what we may be"*
–Hamlet, Act 4, Scene 5

I am more than my body, my torn flesh, my wounded psyche, my aching heart. After waking up from a coma, my initial suffering was related to my physical condition and not being able to move. Then, my emotional and spiritual suffering quickly became the source of my central distress. At times, the enormity of what was happening to me was overwhelming. When I began to look ahead and worry about my future, my suffering was palpable. What value would my life have in the future? I could not see a path beyond my tragedy.

During my final days of my month in the hospital, I required help with my most fundamental needs. I could not wipe myself after a bowel movement. I could not move my legs. I could not hold a spoon. Only by using a pillow for support could I hold a telephone. My mind was engaged but my body was useless. My sense of power-lessness was a great source of suffering, whenever my attention left the moment.

Sometimes I felt like a big baby, needing to be changed and taken care of. This hurt my dignity. A few nurses saw my humanity and interacted with me as one person to another, one nurse to another.

I was deeply lonely. The people in and out of my room all day could not see my inner isolation. Most saw my needs for immediate physical support, nothing more. When people's eyes revealed their sense of empathy for my situation, they rarely spoke about it. Not since my childhood had I felt such loneliness.

I was grateful for my scholarship and research on the subject of suffering, which I had intensely pursued ever since studying Eric Cassell's (1991) book, *The Nature of Suffering and the Goals of Medicine*, in graduate school. Later, I was honored to hear him speak about his work. His insights into suffering helped me see that after I was taken off the ventilator, my suffering was mostly about who I was, not my body, especially since I had no physical pain. Damaged and numb body places left me unable to feel sensations of physical pain, even after five abdominal surgeries. I had no control over anything except my thoughts. Who I had been before cancer had disintegrated in the hospital. Would my integrity ever be restored? After leaving the hospital, who was I to be? What kind of life would I be able to create?

According to Cassell, "suffering is an affliction of the person, not the body" (1999, p. 531). And, "serious illness has an impact on virtually all facets of personhood" (2010, p. 50).

In the hospital and after I came home, I understood that my suffering extended to my personality. Who was I now, after what had happened to me? How would my tragedy affect my social and professional roles with friends, family, and students? Whatever was to become of me?

In the hospital, I was a living case study in suffering. I, the nurse and nursing professor, became the dying patient. The ventilated patient. The patient who awakened with psychosis. The patient whose humanity was hidden inside a broken body. I ached for someone to see beyond my physical struggle, to see and honor my suffering. To compassionately interact with me as a person, not just as a body for interventions.

Before and after I was sick, I taught my students to see beyond their patients' physical suffering to the kind of suffering that cannot be seen without looking for it. I taught them to interact with their patients, one human being to another, at the intersection of hurt and care, fear and compassion. I taught them that, unless they truly understood the nature of suffering, they would never become expert nurses.

CHAPTER 20

VERISIMILITUDE

*"Often times excusing of a fault
doth make the fault the worse by the excuse"*
–King John, Act 4, Scene 2

PART 1

*"If circumstances lead me,
I will find where truth is hid"*
–Hamlet, Act 2, Scene 2

Four days after I left my monthlong hospitalization, an attorney I had called from my hospital bed came to see me at home. Thereafter, we worked together for 2 years, conferring with experts, looking at everything in the medical records provided to us. Still, there were gaps and questions, which only the hospital could answer. It took more than 2 years before the hospital would meet with us. We promised we would not sue; we just wanted to know the truth. Before the hospital meeting, I requested that my surgeons and others read my letter:

> *You want to know what my experience was like? It never occurred to me to go anywhere else for help. I believed in your hospital. Prior to the surgery, I had no diseases, took no medications. I was a healthy woman, except for my cancerous uterus.*

> *I lost my memory for 3 weeks, until I was weaned off the ventilator and experienced severe psychosis, including terror beyond description. During the second surgery to repair my intestine, a faulty intubation caused me irreparable harm, including massive infections, ARDS, and sepsis, all of which required three more surgeries and ventilation for weeks.*

After leaving the SICU, I remained in the hospital for another week and a half, waiting for someone to tell me what had happened. No one came. I felt abandoned and scared. I went home, not knowing what to expect. If someone had explained what I had faced, both physically and psychologically, it would have greatly helped.

I came home with a bag of prescriptions, a bedside toilet, a walker, and a wound vac, attached to a machine I would live with for 2 months. I suffered from high blood pressure, swollen legs, anemia, low-grade fever, night sweats, and post-traumatic stress symptoms that prevented me from sleeping. Someone had to be with me for the next 6 weeks as I could not care for myself. I could not move my legs in or out of bed or carry the wound vac machine. I could not wash my body, or dress myself, or care for my pets. I had no appetite, no joy, and no future. A home health nurse visited me several times a week for more than 2 months. I lost an entire semester of teaching. I lost trust in healthcare and in your hospital.

Fourteen months after leaving your hospital, I had major reconstructive abdominal surgery to repair the 4"× 6" inch hole in my mid-abdomen. I did not choose your hospital—I went elsewhere. I did my best to make sure no resident or fellow or student would make life-and-death decisions about my care. The adhesions inside my body were horrific and complicated. My small intestine had to be resected a second time, because of severe adhesions resulting from major infections and the five surgeries I had endured at your hospital the year before. I suffered the worst pain of my life.

I lost faith—in my body, in your hospital, in my future. I lost my positive body image, my beautiful hair, my smooth abdomen, my vitality, my good health, my independence. I lost time, momentum, and the ability to help others. I lost my abiding sense of well-being.

I continue to be afraid of my body. I'm afraid to lie on my side, afraid of simple movement, of coughing, of developing a hernia, of my damaged lungs getting worse, of adhesions causing discomfort and requiring future surgery, of dying from a heart attack. I'm afraid that I will have to live the rest of my life without the optimism, hope, or sense of equanimity I once had. I'm afraid that I won't have sufficient physical health to be able to do my research, writing, and teaching.

Ultimately, I fear that my death will come from these medical errors, instead of a life naturally lived to its end.

Your hospital failed me. Your surgeons, either inexperienced or distracted, perforated my intestine. You allowed an incompetent student anesthetist to incorrectly intubate me, which caused me to almost die and left me with permanent disability. Nurses were sometimes inept, unkind, and unable to treat me as a human being in distress. The unit I was transferred to after the SICU was often dangerously understaffed.

Other people suffered from my tragedy—my family and friends, my students and colleagues, and my pets. I could not attend to my mother, who was dying and unable to understand where I was or what was happening to me. She died last August. I feel sad when I think of the time I lost with her, including 2 months when I could not see her, much less take care of her.

Two of my sisters, who lived elsewhere, changed their plans and lifestyles to come to the hospital every day to talk with doctors for updates about my hospital situation and to be my advocates.

The worst aspect of my ordeal has been your refusal to explain what happened to me. It would have been much easier for me to accept and adapt to events if you had just told me the truth. No one has ever apologized to me, much less disclosed that errors were made. The traditional institutional culture, which inculcates your staff to delay or deny informing patients of medical errors, must change.

It is my hope that, through exploring and discussing my case, you will improve quality of care for future patients.

From the time I was discharged from the hospital until this meeting, no one ever contacted me or communicated with me in any way, with the exception of my attending surgeon at my scheduled appointments. Before the meeting, my attorney and I never received any information or feedback about my hospital events, other than the medical records we paid to obtain.

Before the meeting, this is what we had learned on our own:

- Day 1: My bowel was damaged by manipulation with non-traumatic graspers, which no one realized until day 3. As toxins infected my body, the delay in diagnosing my torn intestine caused me to develop sepsis, which has a high mortality rate.

- The nurse from my first night in the hospital recognized that my persistent and worsening pain was disproportionate to what was expected after my surgery. Suspecting I had a perforated bowel, she made me NPO (nothing by mouth) in case I went back to surgery.

- Day 2: Seventeen orders and progress notes were written in my chart during an 8-hour period, early in the day, by nine different providers, from at least three different services (Obstetrics, Gynecology, and Gynecologic Oncology), as well as a medical student. Some of these observations, orders, and plans contradicted what others wrote. Yet, no one read these notations or scrutinized the conflicting words. No one was around to oversee the new doctors.

- There was no documentation that anyone ever laid hands on me to touch, palpate, or assess my abdomen, where I had excruciating pain.

- Nothing was documented about me for 5 hours. Nothing to explain why someone (who?) ordered an abdominal X-ray in mid-afternoon. No written assessment of the X-ray results. Were the progress notes missing? Did someone in the hospital destroy written evidence to cover up negligent care, to protect the doctors and the hospital? Or had I simply been left completely alone to die in torment?

- There was a note in my chart (without the time it was written) that stated, "multiple abdominal complaints, hard to examine… will get contrast CT," presumably written around 6 p.m., when the CT scan was ordered.

- Day 3: The CT scan was performed. It showed my perforated bowel. It took 2 more hours before I went to surgery.

- A student was allowed to intubate me incorrectly, causing me to aspirate. Contrast dye in my stomach flooded my lungs, causing chemical burns, pneumonia, and acute respiratory distress syndrome (ARDS), which is associated with a high mortality rate.

- No one—no doctor or surgeon or anyone from anesthesiology—acknowledged or documented witnessing my aspiration during the intubation by the student nurse anesthetist. However, it was noted that a large amount of contrast dye (800–1000 cc) was suctioned from my stomach following the intubation. There was no proof that the attending anesthesiologist was present during the start of my surgery.

- When my attending surgeon wrote my discharge summary a month later, he wrote there was a witnessed (by whom?) episode of aspiration, though there was no such documentation in my chart.

- The botched intubation caused extensive respiratory damage and serious complications, including major bacterial infections throughout my body. Three subsequent surgeries were required to wash out the infection in the membrane (peritoneum) lining my abdominal cavity. This caused significant delay in my recovery. I remained in the hospital for a month.

- I went home with a large, open abdominal wound, attached to a wound vac machine. I needed home health for 2 months and wound care for 6 months, followed by a major surgery a year later to repair the abdominal-wall defects from the previous surgeries.

- At home, I suffered from many physical challenges as well as post-traumatic stress disorder (PTSD) from my prolonged SICU stay on a ventilator, and from the questions and uncertainty surrounding what had happened. I could not return to work until the following year.

- I paid thousands of dollars in medical expenses—for medications and co-pays, food and expenses for caregivers, and expenses for the major reconstructive surgery the following year. I lost months of work and pay. I had permanent scarring, disfigurement, and lung injury.

Before the meeting, we hoped to gain more understanding about events, including: Which surgeon was present at my hysterectomy operation? Who stood right beside my body and controlled the graspers? How much was the new fellow surgeon scrutinized? Why was no one in charge of my post-op care? Why did no one acknowledge my severe pain and intervene? Why did no one comprehend that perforation is the riskiest error that can occur with gastrointestinal surgery? That it can occur in the large or small intestine?

Who exactly was present from anesthesiology at the second surgery? Why did no one realize I had just drunk a gallon of barium dye? Why was a student allowed to intubate me incorrectly, causing extensive lung damage, infections, and three more surgeries?

PART 2

"Tell truth and shame the devil"
—Henry IV, Part I, Act 3, Scene 1

At the hospital meeting, I observed a collection of people, none of whom wanted to be in a small, stuffy, uncomfortable room late on a Friday afternoon; I assumed they already knew it would be a waste of their time. They were not going to tell me anything. They would continue their denial and silence. There was still 1 year left under the statute of limitations for litigation, though I doubt they would have said more if we had waited another year to meet. They were obligated to go through this exercise in futility; it was part of their jobs. I wondered if they had read my letter before the meeting, as requested.

One person seemed neither alert nor interested. If she was attentive, it was difficult to tell; her facial expression was one of boredom and complacency. The risk managers, some of whom were nurses, had some energy. My attending surgeon and the fellow surgeon were present. One of my nurses was there. The certified registered nurse anesthetist (CRNA) who had supervised the student nurse anesthetist was the only person present from anesthesiology. Because I had specifically asked for the student to be present, I asked where he was. I was told that he had moved out of state and could not be found.

Just for the record, I believe I could have found him if I had known his name, but his name was not listed in any of the anesthesia documentation I had twice requested (and twice paid for) from medical records. Nor did the hospital ever reveal his name to me. I could not help but wonder if he was a phantom created to hide the true identity of the person who ruined the intubation.

The hospital administration's position was short and simple: It did nothing wrong. There was no malpractice. No deviation from standards of care. No abrogation of duty. No neglect. No medical errors. They admitted nothing. They expanded on nothing. They were not going to give me any money. It was as though they came to the meeting to see what I knew or thought I knew or how I felt about the situation. They listened like hawks and gave nothing in return.

That evening, I wrote notes from what I heard and understood at the hospital meeting:

- The surgeons made no errors. The graspers were fine. Perhaps my bowel tissue was weak? (i.e., it was my fault my intestine tore). Even though my attending surgeon had documented that in retrospect the graspers were the likely cause of the perforation.

- My horrific post-op pain suggested gas, nothing more. No one would admit—even with 2 years of hindsight and knowing my bowel had in fact been perforated—any errors related to how my level of pain and my vital signs were assessed, interpreted, or monitored the day after surgery.

- My attending surgeon was at an off-site clinic the day after my surgery. There was no one on call or covering my case that day. No one to supervise the nine residents (new doctors) who wrote orders for me to eat breakfast and go home, regardless of my protestations of unbearable pain. The hospital could not refute this, so they simply declared they were unable to name any supervising physician in charge of my case during the day I was dying from a leaking bowel. My attending surgeon was elsewhere in the state, and there was no one providing supervision for the new doctors. Then, no more comment. No explanation. No apology. Of course not—how can you apologize without admitting you did something wrong?!

- There was little to no documentation throughout the day after surgery. Everyone in healthcare knows if something is not documented, it did not happen. The absence of charting is evidence of how poorly I was treated. Or was the documentation incriminating and therefore deleted?

- In spite of my pain, my vital signs were taken only every 4 hours, and then not at all between 3 p.m. and 8 p.m. the day after surgery. If there was any thought that something might be wrong with me, why was I not more closely monitored? I was still there as a patient, even though discharge orders had been written for me to leave that morning. At the very least, a nursing assistant could have regularly taken my vital signs, a task that takes no more than 5 minutes.

- It was not a problem that I had to wait until day 3 to get a CT scan. I was lucky I did not have to wait longer. Amazing!

- Anesthesiology made no errors. The student anesthetist was "excellent" and had performed intubation "hundreds of times." The attending anesthesiologist was "right there." The nurse anesthetist (CRNA) who was at the meeting said, "All of us were right there during the intubation, which was done perfectly. I have never seen one go wrong." I swear to God, that is what he said. Unfortunately, neither my attorney nor I asked, well, if everything was done perfectly, then how come I aspirated?

"And oftentimes, to win us to our harm,
the instruments of darkness tell us truths,
win us with honest trifles,
to betray us in deepest consequence."
–Macbeth, Act 1, Scene 3

After I regained consciousness in the hospital, no one came to discuss my outcomes or complications, however unforeseen and untoward they may have been. This upset me more than anything else. No one ever explained the nature, course, and reason for what went wrong. This left me with questions, concerns, and fears that could have been answered or alleviated with proper attention prior to my discharge. I went home with a broken body and many questions. I had to find my own answers, which took years. This did not have to be.

So, at our meeting, my attorney and I asked the hospital to reconsider how it deals with patients who suffer trauma in the hospital, like I did. They acknowledged they had never considered that patients might suffer trauma after they are admitted. But how could they say they understood? They were never going to admit, "Well, if we screw up and a patient suffers trauma because of our bad care, then we will reconsider how we deal with that."

We asked the hospital to provide additional education to its nurses and residents so they could take better care of critically ill patients who suffer from psychosis and post-traumatic stress disorder. We requested training sessions on the nature of suffering, so nurses, residents, and others could better deal with unexpected complications that cause intensive care unit patients to endure extended stays because of bad outcomes. We urged the hospital to educate its nurses and doctors, as well as risk managers and patient representatives, to tell the patient and family the truth as soon as possible when things go wrong.

"What damned error, but some sober brow
will bless it and approve it with a text"
—The Merchant of Venice, Act 3, Scene 2

I carefully read the hospital's policy regarding disclosure of medical errors resulting in patient injury. It was not followed in my case. Note the distinction between *injury* and *error*:

- As soon as doctors realized I had a perforated bowel and had aspirated in the second surgery, they were required to contact their legal department to receive advice and assistance before giving me or my family any information as to how an *error* occurred, or what issues might have caused said errors. Because this was in the hospital's best interest, this probably happened.

- After my condition had stabilized—which one might say was when I finally left the surgical ICU—my sisters and I should have been promptly told how my *injuries* occurred, including the resulting short- and long-term effects. This did not happen.

- If the hospital determined that errors contributed to my injuries, my family and I should have received a truthful and compassionate explanation about the errors, as well as remedies available to me. This never happened.

- I was to be informed that my injuries would be investigated so other patients would not suffer similar injuries. Then, after the hospital completed its event investigation, I was to receive a full

explanation of any unanticipated outcomes the hospital determined existed in my situation. Unanticipated outcomes sounds
better than medical errors, doesn't it? I was never given any
explanation of confirmed unanticipated or bad outcomes, much
less medical errors or injuries.

- Finally, the hospital's policy required documentation in my
  medical chart—a factual and objective summary describing the
  unanticipated outcomes of my care, and more. If this was done,
  it was either deleted or purposefully omitted from the medical
  chart I paid a lot of money to receive. Since I was supposed to
  have been discharged within 23 hours of my admission, how
  could anyone deny there were unanticipated outcomes when I
  stayed a month?

Before meeting with the hospital, I had little hope for disclosure.
Not after more than 2 years with nothing revealed. Not after all the
back-and-forth communication between my attorney's law firm and
various people in the hospital's legal and risk management divisions.
The hospital knew it was worth the odds to say nothing, to remain
mute, which I am sure was their standard approach. After all, they
were not in court. They did not have to say anything unless a judge
required them under oath to tell the truth. Since I had promised
not to sue, I am certain the hospital planned to keep quiet, in case I
changed my mind.

I chose not to sue because I had already suffered enough, physically
and emotionally, both due to my medical issues and because of the
hospital's treatment of me. Second, a state indemnity statute dictated
that the insurance company would get most if not all of any financial
reward I might win in a legal case. Third, from the beginning, my
attorney's firm had decided not to take my case against the hospital.
They believed they could not win in court. They explained that,
because most juries fail to find the physician or hospital at fault, a
case must be extremely strong to convince a jury that the doctor or
hospital erred.

From the beginning, my attorney had told me she believed most people do not want to believe that medical malpractice is as bad and pervasive as it is, because then they think it might happen to them. That was why, she said, juries tend to support the position of doctors and hospitals, not the patient's case, and why the exceptional cases are ones in which the injuries are so egregious that no one can dispute something went wrong—like when a surgeon amputates the wrong limb.

The best my attorney could hope for was a hospital settlement, from which her firm would get a percentage (usually about one-third) of the award. And, of course, if there was no settlement prior to court, and no adjudication in my favor if we went to trial, the law firm would get nothing. She explained the firm decided it was not worth its time and energy in a culture conditioned to believe the patient is just out for money. Had my leg been amputated instead of my uterus removed, I would definitely have had a stronger case.

I agreed with the law firm. From the beginning, I never wanted to sue. After weighing the risks and benefits, I felt it was not worth it. However, my attorney offered to work with me, *pro bono* (for the public good), to find out the truth, and her firm agreed I would not need to pay her. She thought that once we knew the facts, we could meet with the hospital for clarity and for closure, and that if we promised not to sue, the hospital would be more likely to answer all of my questions and concerns. She was wrong.

I am sure the hospital had closed my case long before the meeting. Even before meeting with me, the hospital had probably memorized its script—there was no wrongdoing, no error, no guilt, no deviation from standards of care, and unless a court deemed otherwise, there was no negligence. There would be no costs for litigation, no increase in malpractice insurance premiums, no money given to me. The hospital was triumphant. I was the only loser.

If the hospital administrators and attorneys learned how to improve medical care from hearing my story, I would never know. How foolish and wrong my attorney and I were, believing our approach might yield fairness and truth. How wrong we were to think the hospital might have behaved with more generosity of openness and goodwill. But, the hospital protectors remained impenetrable. They said nothing. They admitted nothing. If they felt any compassion toward my experience in their business enterprise, they did not let it show.

"A tale told by an idiot,
full of sound and fury,
signifying nothing"
–Macbeth, Act 5, Scene 5

Just before the meeting ended, I expressed my disappointment that, after everything I had been through, not a single person from the hospital had ever said he or she was sorry. The woman who led the meeting immediately turned toward me and said she knew I had been through hell, and she would not trade places with me for anything in the world. This was no apology, though I guess it was something. No one else said a word. She continued, emphatically stating that the hospital would not give me any money. It seemed the hospital wanted to make its final statement on what was most important to them—money. I had not asked for money, just the truth.

Then we all stood up to leave the room. My attending surgeon came around the table with a big smile on his face and hugged me. I am not making this up.

All of my colleagues knew I had been in the hospital for a month and that it was a miracle I had survived. Everyone either encouraged me to sue or asked me why I would not sue. A year before the hospital meeting took place, I had a brief conversation with a colleague who knew about my hospital events. She described her own surgical problems in the same hospital and said they had been very generous in giving her money, and she felt sure they would do the same for me.

I believe the hospital did not offer compensation because that would look like admission of fault. And even though they *were* culpable, they could not take that chance. I think everyone at the meeting had developed a hardened place in their hearts. They needed to protect their sense of decency, justify their silence, and look away from the harm they failed to prevent or acknowledge or make right.

NO ONE IS SAFE WHEN THERE IS SILENCE

"I'll speak to thee in silence"
—Cymbeline, Act 5, Scene 4

I believe that people (doctors, nurses, and others) who work in healthcare do not necessarily pay a higher allegiance to their work than people in other professions. I believe that people who work with excellence and integrity are the exception in any field, while the worst offenders are also the exception; and whether people are mechanics, lawyers, teachers, waiters, or physicians, they all fall along a continuum between the best and the worst.

I believe that just because a person's health, and possibly his or her life, is at stake, it does not mean he or she will necessarily receive a higher order of attention, truthfulness, and excellence than in other situations. I believe that doctors, nurses, and other licensed caregivers are human beings first and healthcare workers second, and all fall prey to the same foibles that affect everyone.

In a hospital, the people who know the truth about work performance include the chief executive officer; administrators in charge of nursing, quality, operations, and finances; medical directors, unit managers, attorneys, and risk managers; human resource directors, department administrators, and members of physician-run ethics committees. The people who run the hospital need to know what goes on in order to manage spending, marketing, and public image. They understand how performance affects the bottom line; their goal is to be financially viable while preserving their reputation.

I believe that transparency is not a given value in the culture of medicine or hospitals, and that it contributes to pockets of silence and ignorance throughout healthcare systems, in which the unsuspecting public puts its trust. I believe that if expert nurses spoke up, without fear of losing their jobs, they would admit that, yes, sometimes doctors deny and nurses cover up for doctors. Without fear of retribution, expert nurses would also tell you that inadequate staffing is a nationwide problem that significantly impacts patient safety.

A few courageous nurses chose not to keep quiet when they decided to speak up for better staffing and safer patient care, as described in an op-ed piece in the *New York Times* (2015) titled "We Need More Nurses," by Alexandra Robbins. In the article, she wrote:

> And yet too often, nurses are punished for speaking out. According to the New York State Nurses Association, this month Jack D. Weiler Hospital of the Albert Einstein College of Medicine in New York threatened nurses with arrest, and even escorted seven nurses out of the building, because during a breakfast to celebrate National Nurses Week, the nurses discussed staffing shortages. (p. A18)

Even though nurses are taught to be the patient's advocate, it is the hospital, not the patient, that provides the nurse with a living wage. It takes a lot of courage to stand up against an employer who holds all the cards.

I believe that medical errors are frequently not revealed or acknowledged; it is impossible to correctly estimate how often errors and adverse events occur, because so many people remain silent or will not tell the truth when things go wrong. How can you collect facts in the absence of transparency?

Hospital personnel know a lot about hidden problems. Most do not blow the whistle; they need their jobs. Doctors are seldom contradicted because there is an assumption that to do so will not accomplish anything. Incompetent doctors are protected by the system and administration, as well as by their patients' fears and ignorance. Some doctors protect themselves with a veneer of self-assuredness, a presumption that they are always right. The really horrific doctors might have to change venue when they lose hospital privileges. Then they go somewhere else, where people once again assume their competence.

When things go wrong in hospitals, patients think what happened to them is an exception. Maybe fate was against them. Or they just had bad luck. They have never heard of a surgeon accidentally nicking an artery. They assume it is a rare event. They are thankful that their doctor saved their life. It is nearly impossible for patients to appreciate their personal story in the greater context of hospital culture across the nation.

Each story is isolated, which protects the doctors and other healthcare providers who may have erred against the patient. A man undergoes a straightforward procedure, but the doctor accidentally cuts his renal artery and he bleeds to death. Does his family ever know? A woman has a mastectomy, but the surgeon accidentally cuts her aorta—she lives. Does the surgeon tell her how it happened? A woman undergoes emergency surgery for appendicitis, but her spinal meningitis goes undetected and she dies. A woman tells the anesthesiologist she is allergic to morphine, but he uses it anyway, either because he forgot or was not paying attention. The woman nearly dies but is resuscitated and lives. Those inside the healthcare world know that there are many thousands of stories just like these.

Sometimes, a rare nurse is brave enough to refuse to be complicit in patient harm and risks her job to do the right thing. A story (later known as the Winkler County nurses whistle-blower case) in the national press in 2009 revealed that two nurses were fired after they wrote a letter to the Texas Medical Board in which they complained about a certain physician's unsafe practices in the county hospital, where the nurses had a combined 47 years of employment. The county sheriff then brought criminal charges against the nurses, which carried potential penalties of 10 years' imprisonment and a maximum fine of $10,000. Charges were dropped against one nurse, while the other nurse endured a 4-day trial and was found not guilty. Ultimately, the doctor pled guilty and was sentenced to 2 months in jail and 5 years of probation. The Winkler County sheriff, county attorney, and hospital administrator ultimately received jail sentences for their roles in trying to silence the nurses (American Nurses Association, 2011).

Sadly, there are few connecting dots from one patient's trauma story to the next, because most errors stay hidden in denial and ignorance. Medical boards (comprised mostly of licensed physicians) protect doctors, and it may be nearly impossible to know if someone has a bad track record. As long as a doctor has a license to practice, one may assume the doctor is good at his or her job, or at least not bad. This is not always true.

An orthopedic surgeon once told me I definitely needed knee surgery and that he might even have to amputate my leg. I immediately left his office and never saw him again, knowing he was wrong. My concern was my health, not pursuing some legal recourse I could not prove or win. It took me 2 months to find a second surgeon, whom I had learned (by asking numerous nurses in the emergency department of the hospital where I worked) was considered to be one of the best orthopedic knee surgeons in my city. When I finally saw him, he said I did not need any surgery.

Years later, someone who worked with the first surgeon—and knew nothing of my association with the practice or the surgeon— revealed to me that there was blatant deceit at the surgery practice; he said there was an effort to create more business (profit) by advising patients to have surgery they did not need. Most patients, he offered, believed anything a doctor told them and, out of fear, hurried to have the recommended surgery.

Standing on my two good original legs, I said nothing. Although I was shocked to hear what this man said, I knew it was true, only because I had the same experience he had described with the same orthopedic practice. Eventually I looked up this surgeon on the state medical licensure site. There was no mention of any problems with him, even though someone I knew had told me he no longer had hospital privileges at a major medical center.

Doctors who fail their patients almost always keep working— because of the deeply entrenched culture of silence inside hospitals, because it takes courage to complain, because dead patients cannot complain, because there are always more unsuspecting patients who know nothing about the doctor's history.

People who work in hospitals know the stories. There are doctors who consistently smell of alcohol and doctors who are too arrogant or doddering to be trustworthy, yet they remain protected. There are arrogant, smug doctors who will not listen to their patients or any-one else, doctors who move away when they lose hospital privileges or reputable standing in the community just to practice somewhere else.

It is time for consumers of medicine to have a realistic understand-ing of the dangers and pitfalls of being a hospital patient, especially in a training institution. When a hospital's first calling is to train its medical staff, patients have no choice but to agree to be guinea pigs or go somewhere else. But there may be nowhere else to go, espe-cially for complicated medical problems. Underling patients, who often have no idea what they are consenting to when they sign on the dotted line, are no match for the powerful healthcare institution.

If you truly want to know who is good at their job, especially a sur-geon, go into the emergency medicine department of a hospital and ask the nurses—they tend to know the truth. Whether or not they reveal it is another matter.

"Cleanse the foul body of the infected world"
—As You Like It, Act 2, Scene 7

It is ironic that hospitals—where people go to get better—harbor harmful microorganisms, invisible murderers of flesh that stalk the halls, rooms, and back closets of our medical institutions. I believe if these microorganisms were visible, hospitals would be run entirely differently.

Some of these organisms, such as *Methicillin-resistant Staphylococcus aureus* (MRSA), *Vancomycin-resistant enterococci* (VRE), and *Clostridium difficile* (C. diff.), kill thousands of people every year. A report in *The New England Journal of Medicine*, based on a 2011 survey of 183 hospitals in 10 states, showed that in that year there were approximately 721,800 infections in 648,000 patients. Roughly 75,000 of these patients died that year as a result of these healthcare-associated infections (Magill et al., 2014).

Additionally, surgical site infections, central-line-associated bloodstream infections, ventilator-associated pneumonia, and catheter-associated urinary tract infections, which occur when invasive procedures and devices are used to treat medical and surgical patients and help them recover, occur in 1 out of every 25 hospitalized patients (Magill et al., 2014).

In March 2016, the Centers for Disease Control and Prevention (CDC) published its healthcare acquired infection (HAI) progress report, based on 2014 data, which includes national as well as state-by-state summaries of six HAI types. This report states that, while there were significant reductions at the national level in 2014, continued prevention efforts are essential to improve patient safety, including changes in state policies. Included in the report is an executive summary, in which the CDC emphasizes that, on any given day, approximately 1 in 25 patients have at least one hospital-acquired infection during their hospital care.

The simplest way to prevent these infections is for medical personnel to wash their hands. Yet, studies continue to reveal that poor hand hygiene in hospitals remains a significant problem due to the poor handwashing compliance of some hospital nurses and doctors. A simple PubMed search on handwashing offers 20 different autofill search options connected to handwashing in healthcare, with more than 6,000 actual results when searching "handwashing" (www.ncbi. nlm.nih.gov/pubmed/?term=handwashing).

How sad that the most dangerous risks in hospitals—surgical errors, medication errors, and infections—are created by the very people who are supposed to heal and protect patients. These professionals, who are obligated to provide skillful, caring, and ethical care, may become a patient's worst enemy. Yet hospitals continue to protect doctors and other healthcare workers, cloaking them in protocol, silence, secrecy, and the language of denial.

Preventing hospital-acquired infections would allow thousands of patients to go home each year instead of going to the morgue.

*"Time shall unfold what plighted cunning hides.
Who covers faults at last with shame derides."*
–King Lear, Act 1, Scene 1

Language can be slippery, especially when used with the intent to protect the guilty. If a doctor could not have reasonably foreseen that his or her actions would harm a patient, then a patient's injuries might be called "unintentional injuries" instead of medical errors. Semantics separate the doctor from the onus of the patient's body. This is just one way hospital administrations (and insurance companies) protect doctors.

If an infection or a surgical error was the *unintended* result of an event, and not the result of a doctor's inattentiveness, carelessness, or poor judgment, then the patient was injured, not by a doctor, but as a result of an event. In my case, I was injured by the nontraumatic graspers, not by the surgeon(s) holding the graspers. If no one *intended* to harm or almost kill you or ruin the rest of your life, your doctor did nothing wrong, however badly things turned out. Doctors are generally not accountable for unintended injuries. Besides, how can anyone prove intent? Bad things happen. Nothing is perfect. There is always risk.

In my situation, the hospital and surgeons had two things in their favor—they did not intend my negative consequences to occur, and I had consented to (my first) surgery. I knew I could not have surgery to remove my cancer unless I signed the hospital's consent form. After the surgical fellow wrote, "Possible laparotomy risks include bleeding, infection and damage to surrounding organs," under the consent form's *Description of the operation or procedure*, I signed, thus sealing my fate to whatever might come. But, I would not have signed if the form had said, "Injury to internal organs might be the result of bad surgery." I would have reconsidered. Even given my fear and intention to swiftly get beyond cancer, I might have chosen another hospital and surgeon. If I had postponed surgery for a few weeks, I would likely have been discharged on day 2, after having just one surgery. I seldom think about this scenario because it is too painful.

When I entered the teaching hospital, covered by my state's health plan, I was the outlier, the outsider, the odd person out. I was not part of the internal alliance of hospital, doctor, and insurance provider. The insurance company's client was the hospital and its doctors, those with whom they regularly did business, not me. Yes, I had cancer and needed surgery, but I was also a part of the medical economy whereby my insurance would help pay the doctors and subsidize the hospital's expenses.

I believe the hospital deemed my injuries unintentional. I do not believe the surgeons in my first surgery intended to injure my small intestine, causing it to later break apart in two places. Nor do I believe the student nurse anesthetist, or anyone else from anesthesiology at my second surgery, intended to almost kill me through aspiration.

Not a single person at the hospital acknowledged anything. Their best course was to stay silent. It was a risk for them to talk, however carefully measured, about anything that might be perceived as a medical error—something that might lead to litigation, that might cost money, that might further compromise their reputation.

If I had gone from coma to death, my bloated, septic corpse would have been wrapped up, placed on the bottom of a hospital bed cart, taken to the morgue, then on to a crematorium. The hospital might have expressed politically correct sympathies to my family, and the silent epidemic of medical errors that involved my death would continue just as they had before.

Throughout my clinical and teaching career, I have heard many stories of medical mishap from people, many of whom did not know I was a nurse or that I had horrific medical stories of my own. Here are a few of the stories shared with me:

- An elderly woman went to the hospital after a severe fall with an obviously broken hand. Even though she repeatedly asked people to do something about it, she was ignored for 10 days. She was then discharged with a permanently bent and impaired hand.

- A clinician tried to pull out a man's catheter without first deflating the internal balloon that holds it in place. This caused the man great pain.

- A woman repeatedly told nurses that she was allergic to the tape they planned to use. They used it anyway. Months later, her injured skin had not healed.

- A severely demented woman periodically lost consciousness. One day when she passed out and fell, hurting her arm in the process, her family took her to the ER. She was discharged a short time later, and no one talked with the family or gave them guidelines for how to prevent these episodes of syncope in the future or when to call 911.

- A man was involuntarily committed by his family members. They were concerned and afraid of the man's violent threats. The hospital decided he was no threat to himself or anyone else and discharged him after a few hours. The man then drove to a family gathering where he shot several people and killed himself.

- After surgery, a woman came to realize that something was physically wrong with her. After repeated office visits for her symptoms, the doctor discovered that a sponge used in her surgery had been accidentally left inside her body.

- A man complained of pain to his urology clinic for years. All he was given was pain medicine. This man's bladder stones went undiagnosed until a doctor new to the practice examined him. Within 5 minutes, the new doctor accurately identified bladder stones as the likely cause of the man's pain. This diagnosis was soon confirmed with a test, and the man had the stones removed.

Unintentional injuries (or death) are caused by doctors (and other clinicians) who lack the intention to harm a patient; such injuries seldom rise to the heinous level of negligible incompetence. But these injuries can cause misery, pain, and suffering, sometimes for the rest of a patient's life.

Injuries (or death) caused by events that should *never* happen are different. *Never events* were first so-named in 2001, by Ken Kizer, MD, a former CEO of the National Quality Forum (NQF), in reference to shockingly inexcusable medical errors that should never occur.

Over time, the list of *never events* has expanded to include adverse events that: (1) are clearly identifiable and measurable, (2) result in death or serious disability, and (3) are usually preventable (Agency for Healthcare Research and Quality, 2014).

By July of 2012, this list included the following seven categories of adverse events (containing a total of 29 examples):

1. Surgical or invasive procedure

2. Product or device

3. Patient protection

4. Care management

5. Environmental

6. Radiologic

7. Potential criminal

A few examples of *never events* include:

- Performing surgery on the wrong site or wrong patient

- Leaving foreign objects inside the patient

- Using contaminated drugs or devices

- Unsafely administering blood

- Causing patient death or serious injury from fall

A well-known *never event* involved hydraulic fluid at a world-renowned medical center where surgical instruments were accidentally washed in the fluid intended for elevator maintenance. These hydraulic-fluid contaminated instruments were then used in surgeries on 3,800 patients (Hoban, 2005).

"If I must die,
I will encounter darkness as a bride,
and hug it in mine arms"
–Measure for Measure, Act 3, Scene 1

A common medical error is misdiagnosis, which leads to delay in treatment. I experienced this as well, when doctors attributed my acute post-op pain only to gas pain, which delayed a CT scan and subsequent bowel repair surgery. While I doubt my surgeons realized my intestine would tear open the night after surgery, my condition could and should have been discovered the following day, at least 24 hours before it was finally identified. But I had no continuity of care after surgery; 2 years later, the hospital could not identify a single physician responsible for my overall care the day after my hysterectomy. My aspiration event was either unknown or denied by the medical team in my emergency repair surgery. It should have been identified before I left the operating room.

Medical errors in hospitals are common and may be divided into categories of error (James, 2013):

1. Errors of commission (errors causing patient harm, like nicking a patient's intestine while removing the gallbladder)

2. Errors of omission (failure to give patient correct test, procedure, or medication)

3. Errors of communication (failing to assess patient for suicidal thoughts)

4. Errors of context (prescribing postdischarge treatment that a patient will be unable to perform)

5. Errors of diagnostics (misdiagnosing and mistreating a patient)

Medication errors are common in hospitals; on average, hospital patients are subjected to at least one medication error per day (Robert Wood Johnson Foundation [RWJF], 2012).

A 5-year study of 10 randomly selected North Carolina hospitals found that "harm resulting from medical care was common, with little evidence that the rate of harm had decreased substantially over a 6-year period ending in December 2007" (Landrigan et al., 2010, p. 2130).

There are many things that can kill you in a hospital, including:

- Bad doctors

- New or inexperienced doctors

- Deadly infection

- Lack of knowledge

- Absence of attention and oversight

- Staff who view you as an object instead of as a suffering human being

- Poor or no critical-thinking skills

- Absence of coordinated care

- No timely follow-up

- Poor or no communication

- Unsafe practice

All of the above applied to me, and whether or not you die from the harm, you or your family will probably never know what went wrong.

"Once more unto the breach"
–Henry V, Act 3, Scene 1

A doctor is late and hurries into the room to circumcise a new-born infant. To the horror of nurses and other people watching, he proceeds to cut off the foreskin without first giving the infant pain medicine. While his observers know he is violating policy, that he is making up for his tardiness by failing to provide adequate care for his patient, they say nothing. Noting their facial expressions, he brusquely dismisses it in light of the child's age, saying that the baby will not remember the pain.

Whatever circumcision technique the doctor used, he most certainly separated part of the penis from underlying tissue, then crushed the tissue with a clamp as he cut away the foreskin and then left the clamp in place long enough (5 minutes or so) for blood to coagulate. A student who was present at this circumcision told me this story, and it made me angry. I was personally going to file a complaint until I learned that it took place in another hospital in a nearby city.

An operating room nurse steals clear liquid pain medication out of vials and then refills them with water. He then assists in surgeries with patients who receive water instead of pain medicine. He knows the patients are in pain and unable to understand or communicate what is happening. I worked with this man, a former opiate addict, and he told me this story.

A parent insists, privately, to the nurse and doctor that she does not want her adolescent child to have the prescribed narcotic, even if it is indicated. The patient does not get pain relief and continues to suf-fer and never knows why. A nurse told me this story.

A nurse routinely refuses to give ordered prn (as needed) pain medication to patients with histories of addiction, as a way of punishing them for past bad behavior. Multiple nurses have told me stories of this nature.

JUSTICE

"Time is the justice that examines all offenders"
—As You Like It, Act 4, Scene 1

Only with our legal system is there hope for justice. Without the law, there is no hope. Hospitals spend millions of dollars on malpractice insurance and their legal and risk management departments. These experts know exactly how to state their standard-of-care policies to disallow legitimate claims of medical malpractice.

Profit is almost always the prevailing motivation of corporations, including hospitals and universities. What if hospitals put as much time, energy, and money into preventing medical errors as they did into financing their legal and risk management teams and insurance companies? Would they save money?

I believe that a top priority in many hospitals is to deny and delay disclosure regarding medical wrongdoing and thus stave off potential medical malpractice claims, even if the hospitals realize they may eventually have to go to court. I believe that hospitals work hard to keep their funds as long as possible, even if they believe they will eventually have to settle a case. I believe hospitals will only settle a malpractice claim if they believe the claim is undeniably true and egregious, if a trial seems inevitable, and if going to trial is more expensive than a settlement out of court.

For a patient to successfully win a malpractice claim against his or her doctor, the patient must show that the physician rendered negligent care, and the negligent care injured the patient. For a successful malpractice action, these four legal elements must be proven:

1. A professional duty was owed to the patient

2. A breach of such duty occurred (deviation from standard of care)

3. Injury was caused by the breach

4. Resulting damages

If awarded, monetary damages are usually based on both actual economic loss and noneconomic loss, such as pain and suffering (Bal, 2009).

While most U.S. physicians will face a malpractice lawsuit at some time in their careers, a major 2011 study that provided a most comprehensive risk analysis for malpractice claims by physician specialty found that the annual chance of a claim varies from around 5% in low-risk specialties to nearly 20% in specialties at the highest risk (Jena et al., 2011).

Was there a breach of duty in my initial surgery? I will never know. Did my attending surgeon properly oversee and assist the new fellow to properly manipulate my organs with long instruments stuck through the tiny holes they made into my body? It was August—the new fellow had just arrived at the hospital for the next phase of his surgical training. Had this new surgeon ever observed or participated in my type of surgery? Had he handled the type of graspers used in my laparoscopic hysterectomy? Did my attending surgeon violate a standard of care by allowing a neophyte to put me in harm's way? Would another teaching surgeon have shown and explained to the new surgeon—there to observe—how to properly grasp and hold an intestine out of the way for the harvesting of lymph nodes?

My attending surgeon never told me who held which grasper and for how long, and for what purpose. He never explained if he could tell how much pressure the new fellow applied as he grasped my small intestine. He only said that neither of them realized my bowel had been injured during the surgery.

Unfortunately, the great tragedy was that no one supervised my care the night after surgery, or the following day. This caused a significant and potentially deadly delay in diagnosis and treatment. I believe that when the doctors failed to provide proper post-op care for me, they breached their duty. There was no doctor to guide the new residents in how to correctly evaluate my pain, order a CT scan in a timely fashion, or get me to lifesaving surgery as soon as possible.

On day 3, during the emergency surgery to repair my bowel, there were more breaches of duty: when a student was allowed to intubate me incorrectly; when no one recognized and documented my aspiration caused by the failed intubation; when no one immediately provided care to prevent and mitigate any resulting infections or other injuries. Because of the student's failure to properly intubate me and the surgical team's failure to recognize and treat my aspiration, I suffered three more surgeries and weeks on a ventilator.

A doctor is legally at fault for medical malpractice when the doctor fails to provide the quality of care required by law. How quality of care is determined is crucial to this point. To prevail in court, the doctor must demonstrate that minimally sound judgment was used to give minimally competent care. If my case had gone to court, I do not believe anyone could have justifiably proved I received minimally competent care, not when what was supposed to be 1 day turned into a month, and one surgery turned into five.

I wonder how hospitals rationalize preventable hospital medical errors and adverse events. Surely many malpractice claims must relate to these preventable errors. What would happen if hospitals and healthcare insurance companies valued transparency and if doctors and nurses valued truth-telling? Would there be less injury and less law, with more cure and care in medicine?

A BETTER FUTURE

"Men at some time are masters of their fates.
The fault, dear Brutus, is not in our stars
but in ourselves, that we are underlings."
–Julius Caesar, Act 1, Scene 2

Hospitals are corporations. Even if described as nonprofit or not-for-profit, make no mistake that money is very important to them. Financial health is important, but it should not be more important than providing excellent patient care. Money should not be the determining factor in whether a hospital and its doctors discover and disclose and learn from their preventable medical errors.

How much money would a hospital ultimately save if it trained nurses and residents to understand and identify ethical dilemmas? To see and ameliorate suffering? What if a hospital's highest priority was to build cooperation, coordination, and collaboration among its doctors and nurses so they could all work together for their patients' highest well-being? What if hospitals and the doctors and nurses who worked there were united in their resolve to use the truth about medical errors to improve the system for everyone?

How long will hospitals (and their insurance companies) value money over ethical conduct? How long will nurses and doctors be too afraid to tell the truth when things go wrong? How long will it take for transparency to become a valued goal in healthcare?

Is it possible that a hospital environment of transparency might actually cost the hospital less than its machinations of long-standing institutional silence? I believe when people truly understand what goes on in hospitals, the tide will turn, the dots will connect, and there will no longer be pockets of silence. Perhaps healthcare consumers—the patients and families—will be the guiding force in transforming the hospital paradigm.

*"There is a tide in the affairs of men
which taken at the flood leads on to fortune;
omitted, all the voyage of their life
is bound in shallows and in miseries.
On such a full sea are we now afloat,
and we must take the current when it serves,
or lose our ventures."*
–Julius Caesar, Act 4, Scene 3

There are many excellent nurses and physicians working on behalf of patients throughout our country's healthcare system. Yet, it is inevitable that sometimes they will fail their patients. Even in the best-run hospitals, medical errors and adverse events occur.

While it is unreasonable to hope for no errors, it is reasonable to hope that, when these errors occur, people will tell the truth, especially so they can learn how to prevent future errors. A hospital's highest priority should be to provide excellent patient care, which is only possible if preventable medical errors and adverse events are acknowledged and eradicated.

Each of us has a stake in better healthcare, for ourselves and for those we love. In a world that sometimes seems to be corrupt and beyond redemption, there is still much we can accomplish on a smaller scale. We can decide to change how we view and treat patients. We can choose to learn and work together. We can pledge to value the role of each medical professional. We can create horizontal leadership.

Intention is a universal guiding force. Our actions flow from our integrity. We can choose which moral and ethical principles guide our professional practice. We can commit to put the patient's highest safety and good above all else; to honor the patient's autonomy, ensuring the patient's right to know the truth and choose or refuse treatment; to practice beneficence by putting the patient's best interest first; to use resources fairly and competently, creating the greatest good for the most people; to see and address suffering, wherever we find it; and to respect the personhood and dignity of each patient, as well as each nurse, doctor, and any healthcare worker who serves the patient.

If we intend to change, we can provide better care. If we intend to tell the truth, we can operate with transparency. With knowledge and imagination, we can transform our healthcare system into a better model for patients and practitioners. We can learn to practice compassion for everyone, including ourselves, as we work together to be wiser and more conscious.

Our destiny is not in the stars, but in ourselves.

EPILOGUE

"Action is eloquence"
–Coriolanus, Act 3, Scene 2

For many years, I regularly asked myself what my purpose was in being alive. Yes, I was good person, a dutiful citizen. I cared about others. I tried to do what was right. I did my best, as a friend, sister, daughter, nurse, and teacher. But was that enough? I seemed not to think so. I was not raising children or inventing something to improve people's lives. My daily activities were nothing unique. That all changed the weekend I woke up in the SICU with absolutely no idea where I was or what had happened to me. Instinctively and immediately, I knew that my story was important and worth writing.

Perhaps forming the will to live—so I could tell my story—was the earliest indicator that I would not give in to the hopeless despair that overwhelmed me in my immobile body. I had to survive; I needed to be alive to learn the facts and put the pieces together. As I went through the days, weeks, and months that followed, I never wavered in my resolve to write this book. I was no longer asking the universe why was I here; I now knew.

In my quest to uncover my hospital story, I never imagined I would come to see our healthcare system as broken as it is. Realizing how many hospitals are influenced by machinations of ignorance and greed has been disheartening, though I have no doubt improvement is possible. Even though I trust less and question more, I have compassion for those who stand in the way of the safety and sanctity of patients. I also believe change will come as people learn more and stop accepting the old status quo.

My physical recovery has taken years and is still ongoing. I have been able to regain some of the function I thought might be forever lost. As for my psyche, instead of asking daily why am I here, I now ask: Where is my moral life expanding, and how can I make a positive difference in the lives of others?

Living in compassion is often as easy as breathing. I forgive more easily and more quickly. I have less anger and more patience. Through my hospital experiences of suffering, I feel more connection with other people, especially my patients. Love may not always bind us, but suffering surely does. I also remember that the most important aspects of character are invisible: courage, resilience, curiosity, respect, tolerance, and kindness.

Here are a few pointers in how to take care of yourself when you enter a healthcare system:

Become your personal medical consumer advocate:

- Pay attention, even if you must detach from your emotions as a patient.

- Ask questions and take notes.

- Remain skeptical and alert.

- Identify your assumptions and validate them.

- Never assume you are being told what you most need to know, much less all you need to understand.

- Make sure you or someone with you knows what medication you are prescribed and given, and for what purpose. Remember that medication errors are common in hospitals. Realize that you may refuse medication for any reason.

- Whenever possible, have someone act as your advocate and witness.

- Learn as much as possible about your health issues so you can formulate relevant questions and concerns to share with your physician or other caregivers.

- Realize and remember that sickness and treatment are about much more than a physical problem, disease, or trauma: They are also about suffering, fear, anxiety, loneliness, support, and hope.

After you receive bad health news:

- When you hear bad news, do not necessarily assume it is true. It might be, but become your personal devil's advocate. Do not allow fear to be your driving force. It is not unusual for a second opinion to yield a different diagnosis. A second opinion may be essential to confirm a correct diagnosis and, as well, may give you more treatment options for consideration. Always get a second opinion.

- Ask other people—a neighbor, colleague, friend, family member, or someone from your religious community or groups of interests—if they know anything about your diagnosis. When I asked people about uterine cancer, several people told me there was a high success rate with surgery, assuming the cancer had not spread. This immediately gave me hope.

- Find out which doctor has the reputation for being the best person to help you, but remain skeptical—even bad doctors have fans. If you personally know people who work in health-care, such as a nurse or physician, ask them who they would go to—and why—if they received your diagnosis.

- If you have more than one hospital to choose from, learn how various hospitals deal with your problem. For example, breast cancer treatments vary widely depending on where you live and which hospital you choose.

- The Internet provides comprehensive information about most anything; make sure you use only reliable sources—websites such as MedlinePlus from the U.S. National Library of Medicine, WebMD, Sharecare, or the Mayo Clinic. Unscientific blogs may confuse or alarm you as it is difficult to verify their stories or claims.

- Finally, remember that knowledge is power. Learning about your health crisis may not only guide your choices, it may also empower you with a sense of control during a time when life feels scary.

Before you go to an outpatient treatment center or into a hospital:

- If possible, have your affairs in order, especially your legal will and your advance directives—living will and healthcare power of attorney. Prepare for the worst scenario and hope for the best outcome. Take copies of your advance directives with you when you go for treatment. Also, tell your friends and family what they might need to know in case you do not come home on schedule, or worse.

- Make arrangements for your home, pets, mail, and other matters you will not be able to attend to while out of commission.

- Items you may need include personal telephone, watch or clock, pen and paper, contact information for people you might need to talk with, and reading material—preferably something that inspires you.

- Make sure you tell your loved ones ahead of time how you feel about visitors—which ones and how often. Since I planned to be home about 24 hours after entering the hospital, I expected to have no visitors, only the friend who was with me. Later, my family knew I would not want visitors while I was in a coma.

While you are in the hospital:

- Have someone with you as much as possible—someone who is not afraid to ask tough questions or speak up if something does not seem right, someone who can help make decisions (or call the right people) if something goes wrong. Choose a person who is brave enough to risk being seen as inappropriate or meddling. It is better to appear foolish than to risk saying nothing, in case something is not right. There is nothing more important than your physical and emotional well-being when you are under the control of a medical system.

- If your doctor or nurse (or someone else) is not giving you the right care or is not treating you with respect, ask to speak with someone in authority, such as the nursing unit manager, the nursing supervisor, the doctor's supervisor, or the administrator in charge. If you do not know how to contact any of these people, pick up the telephone and dial the operator for assistance. I once knew a woman whose arms had been severely injured, leaving her unable to wipe herself in the bathroom. When I learned that a nurse was not helping her with that chore, I spoke to the unit manager to insist the nurses perform correctly.

- If you cannot get the nutrition you need, ask someone to bring you food you can eat.

- In general, do not be afraid to ask for anything that might help you, even if you think your request cannot be met. You never know. And, if you cannot speak for yourself, make sure you have a personal advocate who can look after your needs. Staffing shortages are common in hospitals.

DO YOU HAVE A STORY?

Do you have a story of surviving preventable medical errors or adverse medical events? Or do you know someone affected by, or who died from, medical errors or adverse medical events?
If so, please send the story to Donna Helen Crisp at thepatientinroom2@gmail.com.

GLOSSARY

Acute respiratory distress syndrome (ARDS): A lung condition in which fluid replaces oxygen in your air sacs and you cannot breathe. Mortality is 26–58%. Older patients have a higher risk of dying. People who develop ARDS are usually in the hospital for serious health problems that might not necessarily involve their lungs.

Advance directives: Legal documents you create (no need for an attorney) and notarize to indicate your wishes if you cannot communicate in a healthcare crisis. A *living will*—sometimes described as a declaration of desire to die a natural death—instructs healthcare providers when to withhold or withdraw life-prolonging measures in certain situations. A *healthcare power of attorney* names one or more persons to speak for you if you are unable to communicate; providers choose the first person listed and only go to others on the list, in order, if the first person is unable or unwilling to be your advocate.

Autonomy: The principle that adults have the legal and ethical right to participate in decisions about their own health care and to maintain the personal choice and right to say "yes" or "no" to medical interventions. Autonomy also includes the right not to participate in decision-making or to delegate this process to someone else.

Beneficence: The ethical principle, intention, and practice of doing what is right and good to benefit the patient.

Checklist, the: When Peter Pronovost, MD, PhD, FCCM, of Johns Hopkins Medicine and Johns Hopkins University School of Medicine, began to study healthcare- or hospital-acquired infection (HAI) in 2001, he determined that five simple steps, if followed by doctors, would greatly reduce infections when inserting a central venous catheter (central line)—a catheter that is placed into a large vein, commonly in a patient in the emergency department or intensive care unit (ICU). In 2007, Atul Gawande wrote an article that was published in *The New Yorker* and titled "The Checklist," which described Pronovost's five simple steps: 1) Wash hands with soap; 2) clean the patient's skin with chlorhexidine antiseptic; 3) put sterile drapes over the entire patient; 4) wear a sterile mask, hat, gown, and gloves; and 5) put a sterile dressing over the catheter site. Gawande went on to describe the Keystone Initiative in Michigan, when hospitals began using Pronovost's checklist in their intensive care units to insert a central line catheter into a patient's large vein. Using this checklist caused the infection rate to drop by 66%—to such a low level that the Michigan hospital ICUs outperformed 90% of intensive care units nationwide. Preventable infections in hospitals and other healthcare facilities constitute a major patient-safety hazard. If more checklists were mandatory throughout healthcare settings, including all emergency departments and ICUs, there would be fewer mistakes, fewer deaths, and enhanced patient safety.

Certified registered nurse anesthetist (CRNA): A master's prepared, advanced practice nurse who works as part of the anesthesiology team in operating room surgery.

Coma, medically induced: An induced state of deep consciousness, maintained by medications, so the patient can have surgery and/or be maintained on a ventilator.

Computerized tomography (CT) scan: A series of x-rays taken from different angles that are then processed into cross-sectional images (slices) of bones, blood vessels, and soft tissues. A CT scan is particularly useful in examining a patient who might have unknown internal injuries, such as a perforated bowel.

Deconditioned body: Inactivity from staying in a hospital bed (or being in a coma) that causes reduced functional capacity and negative symptoms in multiple body systems, especially the musculoskeletal system. Deconditioning is commonly caused by multiple trauma, orthopedic injury, stroke, prolonged hospitalization, or heart attack. A total lack of activity for 3 to 5 weeks can cause a 50% reduction of muscle strength.

Dehydration: When you use or lose more fluid than you take in, causing your body to have insufficient water and other fluids for normal bodily function. Causes include exercise, diarrhea, vomiting, fever, and excessive sweating. Signs of dehydration include dry mouth, fatigue, thirst, decreased urine output, headache, constipation, and lightheadedness. Severe dehydration can become a medical emergency.

Endotracheal (ET) tube: A tube inserted though the mouth or nose into the trachea (windpipe) to establish and maintain a patient's airway and to ensure that there is an adequate exchange of oxygen and carbon dioxide.

Ethics, medical: Moral principles relevant to values and judgments in the medical environment. Beneficence (doing good) and nonmaleficence (not doing harm) must be balanced. An injection might sting, but the higher good is pain relief or disease resistance from a vaccination. Autonomy and the patient's right to self-determination are valued but are sometimes in conflict with what the doctor wants to do (paternalism). Other medical ethical concepts include respect for human rights, justice (allocation of resources), confidentiality, and informed consent (which might or might not sufficiently inform the patient). Euthanasia, assisted suicide, transplants, fertility, and abortion are often ethically framed by those with various beliefs.

Fidelity: An ethical principle that honors the importance of the relationship between the patient and caregiver. Through keeping one's commitment and promise to the vulnerable patient—to care for the patient and maintain confidentiality—a nurse or doctor demonstrates loyalty by creating and maintaining trust with the patient. Sharing the patient's information with a treatment team does not breach confidentiality.

Hair thinning or loss (telogen effluvium): *See* telogen effluvium.

Hallucinations: Perceptions created by your mind that involve one or more of your five senses and seem real but are not. Examples include seeing spiders or hearing voices that are not there. Common causes include mental illness, substance abuse, and delirium.

Healthcare- (or hospital-) acquired infection (HAI): Preventable infections that patients acquire while being treated for other conditions. These infections, often associated with the use of a central line, catheter, or ventilator, can be drug-resistant bacteria that are hard or impossible to eradicate, including Methicillin-resistant *Staphylococcus aureus* (MRSA), Vancomycin-resistant *Enterococci* (VRE), and *Clostridium difficile* (C. diff.). Acute care infections can be categorized into four major categories: 1) surgical site infections, 2) central line–associated bloodstream infections, 3) ventilator-associated pneumonia, and 4) catheter-associated urinary tract infections. In 2016, the Centers for Disease Control and Prevention published the results of a project known as the HAI Prevalence Survey, which found that HAIs reported in 2011 included an estimated 722,000 HAIs in patients in U.S. acute care hospitals, of whom about 75,000 died during their hospitalizations.

Hopelessness: When sick patients expect a negative outcome and believe they lack power to change their situation, they become hopeless. Hopelessness can compromise the immune system and increase a person's chance of getting heart disease or cancer. Hopelessness can also lead to depression, especially if the person no longer has interest in or enjoys normal activities.

Hospitalist: A doctor employed by the hospital or other acute care setting to organize care for hospitalized patients. The hospitalist, generally a doctor the patient has never met, oversees the patient's care. Patients cannot choose which hospitalist sees them, and they often have a new doctor each week. Patients over age 65, often with a lengthy health history that includes chronic medical conditions, make up the largest group of patients in acute care settings. No matter how experienced and caring a hospitalist might be, this type of doctor has no sense of the patient's complex history (personal and medical) and must start over with assessment and communication, depending heavily on what might be in a patient's electronic record.

A patient's hospitalist and surgeon have much in common; often, they have never seen the patient before the current medical problem. They know little of the patient's personhood, including the patient's personal and emotional history. And, after they perform their role in the patient's current health dilemma, they typically never see that patient again, except for brief office follow-up or future care with similar issues.

Iatrogenesis: From the Greek for "brought forth by the healer," this term refers to the unintended adverse consequences a patient experiences in a hospital, including medical errors; negligence; infection; drug interactions; or unprofessional treatment from a nurse, doctor, pharmacist, or others.

Informed consent: A legal document signed by the patient giving the provider permission to perform surgery, treatment, interventions, or other patient care. When a teaching hospital's mission to train its medical staff trumps its commitment to provide the highest quality care, informed consent may be the ultimate symbol of the unfortunate disparity between what is best for the surgeon, new or seasoned, and what is best for the patient. Unless it is an emergency situation, a patient (or designated friend or family member) must give consent before treatment takes place.

Intensive care unit (ICU): A hospital unit where patients with severe and life-threatening illnesses or injuries are closely monitored by nurses and doctors who intensively treat patients using technology, special equipment, and medications.

Intubation: Procedure whereby a flexible plastic tube is inserted into a patient's windpipe for the purpose of maintaining an open airway or administering certain medications.

Justice: Justice means fairness. In a healthcare setting like a hospital, where providers attend to multiple patients, it is important that each patient has his or her needs met—while providers consider all patients in terms of the resources of staff, time, and other factors.

Providers need to balance what is best for one patient with what is best for all patients.

Laparoscopic surgery: Minimally invasive surgical technique in which small incisions are made in the body, and instruments are then put through those openings to conduct the surgery. This surgery has a shorter recovery time than regular surgery, but it does not allow for direct observation of what is inside the body.

Liability: A legal obligation one is required to fulfill.

Litigation: A lawsuit or legal action to determine legal rights and remedies of the person involved in a dispute. In medical malpractice, litigation usually involves both doctor and patient.

Medical error: A preventable adverse outcome from care, whether evident or harmful, to the patient. Examples include misdiagnoses; unnecessary tests, treatments, and procedures; erroneous treatments; medication errors; injuries from falls and immobility; inappropriate blood transfusions; central line infections, catheter–associated urinary tract infections; bedsores (skin breakdown); surgical site infections; blood clots; ventilator-associated infections; uncoordinated care; missed warning signs (vital signs, pain); poor or absent communication; pharmacy errors; lab errors; and birth injuries.

Mindfulness: Being aware, in the present moment, without judgment.

Moral distress: A serious problem in nursing that causes nurses to lose a sense of integrity and satisfaction with their work environment. Studies have shown that moral distress is a major factor for nurses leaving a work setting or the profession.

Nasogastric (NG) tube: A narrow tube passed through the nose into the stomach, commonly used to provide liquid nutrition or to aspirate stomach contents.

Never events: Shocking medical errors that should never occur. Categories include surgical, product, or device; patient protection; care management; environmental; radiologic; and criminal. Examples include food inserted into the chest tube instead of the stomach tube; air bubbles going into an IV catheter, resulting in a stroke; sponges, wipes, scissors, and other instruments left inside a patient's body after surgery; amputation of the wrong limb.

Nonmaleficence: This ethical principle means *do no harm*. Sometimes risks and benefits must be weighed to determine how to give the best patient care with the least harm. For example, the benefit of receiving an injection may outweigh the few seconds of pain from the needle or minor side effects of the treatment.

Nosocomial: Literally means originating in a hospital. Typically used to describe infections patients acquire after they are admitted to a hospital.

Paternalism: From the Latin word for "father," paternalism in healthcare usually refers to a doctor (or some other provider) who believes his or her expertise and opinion take priority over what the patient might want, assuming there is discussion. Paternalism is the opposite of self-determination. Historically, patients believed and trusted, with little or no discussion, that the doctor would look out for their best interest and do what was right. The paternalistic doctor was like a father figure, who often knew the patient well and certainly knew more than the patient did about health matters. Medical knowledge was a hard-earned asset, and patients and families revered the physician because that knowledge was generally not available to them. Patients now have a world of information at their fingertip and can, and should, seek answers to all their questions and concerns—not just acquiesce to a medical provider's authority without adequate reasoning.

Peritonitis: Can result from a rupture in the abdomen, causing an inflammation of the peritoneum—the thin membrane lining the inner abdominal wall and covering organs inside the abdomen.

Post-traumatic stress disorder (PTSD): This disorder was first formalized in 1980 after 58,220 U.S. military personnel died and more than 150,000 were wounded in the Vietnam War. People with PTSD suffer from flashbacks, nightmares, intrusive thoughts, and severe anxiety—often for the rest of their lives. These symptoms make up a difficult mental health disorder caused by a terrifying event in the past, either witnessed or experienced.

Powerlessness: Hospital patients might feel powerless over a situation, believing that they have no personal power to control events, environment, or destiny. This feeling leads to a sense of hopelessness and possibly depression.

Psychosis: A severe mental disorder in which a person has a break from reality and can suffer with impaired thoughts and emotions that distort external reality.

Risk management: A complex process of identifying, assessing, and averting risks throughout hospitals. The ultimate goals are to maximize patient and institutional safety, comply with federal regulations, prevent potential risks, and maintain legal soundness by preventing, mitigating, or minimizing harm and unsafe practices.

Self-determination: Individuals have the right to determine what happens to them. In healthcare settings, a patient might willingly relinquish self-determination to a doctor (or other provider) to make decisions.

Sepsis: A life-threatening condition, sepsis usually stems from an inflammatory response to infections in the abdomen, lungs, kidneys, or bloodstream. Mortality rate is 40–60%, with elderly people having the highest risk of death.

Suffering: The state of undergoing pain, distress, or hardship. Suffering may be obvious in someone who is in physical pain. Suffering that is mental, psychological, or spiritual, however, is not always visible. No external clues may exist for others to notice internal suffering, which must be believed to be seen. Excellent clinicians "assume" that every patient is suffering in some way. This does not mean every patient wants or needs to share his or her suffering with a nurse or other provider. It does mean that nurses and doctors who "know" a patient is suffering are more likely to see the patient as a person and not just a body. Other words for suffering include adversity, anguish, discomfort, distress, misery, and torment.

Telogen effluvium (hair thinning or loss): The sudden, unexpected loss of hair caused by severe mental stress or by major illness, surgery, high fever, or severe infection.

Trauma: A deeply disturbing experience—psychological, physical or both—in which a person is injured, damaged, or wounded in some way. Common examples include car accidents, sudden death of loved ones, and serious complications from hospital medical care.

Uterine and endometrial cancer: Uterine cancer starts in the muscle layer or supporting connective tissue of the uterus. Most cancers of the uterus begin in the cells of the inner lining (endometrium) of the uterus and can spread locally to the cervix and other parts of the uterus. It can also spread regionally to nearby lymph nodes, which are small, pea-sized organs that are part of the body's immune system. In addition, the cancer can spread to lymph nodes in the pelvis along the aorta (the main artery from the heart down to the back of the abdomen and pelvis). If untreated, the cancer can spread (metastasize) to distant lymph nodes, upper abdomen, and omentum (the large fatty sheet of tissue in the abdomen that spreads over the stomach, intestines, and other organs) or to other organs, including the lung, liver, bone, and brain.

Ventilator: A medical machine that mechanically moves breathable air in and out of the lungs to provide the mechanism of breathing for a patient who is physically unable to breathe or unable to breathe enough.

Veracity: This ethical principle relates to truth-telling. The caregiver is accurate and faithful to the facts. Veracity is grounded in respect for the patient's right to know the truth and make decisions accordingly (patient autonomy). Veracity does not mean always telling the patient everything. Patients who practice autonomy (self-determination) may choose what they do or do not want to know.

Vipassana: Insight into the true nature of reality, achieved by being mindful of one's breathing, thoughts, feelings, and actions. One might say that "vipassana" is the extreme opposite of psychosis.

READER'S GUIDE

DISCUSSION QUESTIONS & ETHICAL EXPLORATIONS

Use the following discussion questions and ethical exploration prompts to consider the author's experience of surviving trauma caused by preventable medical errors.

MEDICAL CARE

The following medical care questions are directed toward healthcare students or staff but may be of interest to all readers.

Informed Consent

1. The author of this book was diagnosed with uterine cancer. Her surgeon recommended laparoscopic surgery—also called minimally invasive surgery—to remove her uterus and harvest lymph nodes for cancer biopsy through the use of instruments inserted into tiny incisions in her body. After she recovered from her medical ordeal, she learned that she may not have been the best candidate for a laparoscopic hysterectomy. Had she better understood the risks of laparoscopy, she might have chosen general surgery. What kinds of surgery are commonly done laparoscopically? What are the advantages, disadvantages, and risks of laparoscopy versus general surgery? The use of computer-assisted robots is increasingly common in surgeries that were once done laparoscopically. In this surgical approach, a surgeon, with the help of a computer program, controls tiny tools attached to a robotic arm. Consider and discuss if using a robot to perform surgery might increase or decrease patient safety.

2. What are the basic elements of informed consent? Are there inherent conflicts in how informed consent serves the patient, doctor, and hospital? Was the author fully informed as to the risks and benefits of the surgery for which she consented? Consider and discuss a scenario that facilitates fully informed consent.

3. Later in the book (Chapter 15), as the author prepared for reconstructive surgery, she requested specific changes to the consent form. At first, the anesthesiologist resisted her request. After pursuing the matter through the hospital's risk management team, via her pre-op nurse, she was allowed to make her requested changes. The author was proactive, having thought carefully about what she would and would not agree to prior to surgery. How many patients (and nurses and doctors) realize a patient has the right to request changes to an informed consent form before signing? Does your organization have procedures for special requests related to informed consent? As your patient's advocate, how would you handle such a situation?

Preventable Errors

1. After the author's hysterectomy, she was returned to her room to recover before her planned release the next morning. Review her description (in Chapter 3) of her post-surgical care, particularly how the providers addressed her ever-increasing pain. No one supervised the new residents who were responsible for her post-op care. How did this affect the residents' critical thinking skills? How did their inexperience affect their assessment skills? What factors did they fail to consider regarding her pain?

2. While pain is often considered the fifth vital sign, many physicians consider pain to be a symptom, not a vital sign, since pain cannot be measured in the same manner as heart rate,

respiratory rate, temperature, and blood pressure. Why did the doctors fail to adequately assess and address her pain? Why did they fail to seriously consider her verbal concerns?

3. The use of carbon dioxide gas—to inflate the abdominal area to allow for visibility during laparoscopic surgery—is common. It is unlikely, or impossible, for this gas to cause death. Given that bowel perforation is perhaps the most serious complication of any gastrointestinal surgery—and is considered to be an emergency complication that will result in death if not addressed—why did the doctors focus only on gas pain? Have you ever considered that postoperative care may present more risks than the surgery itself?

4. The author suffered a cascade of preventable medical errors—both in action and in omission—during her medical saga, which took place in a teaching hospital in late summer, when residents are still new and inexperienced. Two years later, the hospital admitted that, on the day following the first surgery, the residents were not attended by an experienced surgeon. How might an experienced surgeon have taught the residents how to assess the author's pain and ensure she was safely cared for? Discuss the value of hands-on experience versus academic learning. How can novice doctors make the transition to expertise without compromising patient care? Can this learning curve occur in a way that does not compromise patient safety?

5. The author suffered for an unconscionably long time with her surgically induced injury before her medical team ordered a CT scan to investigate the potential cause of her pain. Review Chapter 4 and discuss the point in her care when—given your understanding of *standards of care*—someone from her surgical team should have ordered a scan to rule out internal injury. Write a short paragraph or list detailing the steps, and timing of steps, on the day she was to go home that might have prevented some or all of her future harm in subsequent surgeries.

6. After the scan revealed the author's injury, she was rushed into surgery to repair her damaged bowel, only to suffer additional medical injuries—the most serious being the damage to her lungs during anesthesia. When a student who was allowed to intubate her used the wrong technique to anesthetize her for surgery, she suffered what she considered to be the most egregious and damaging consequence of all her surgeries. Was it ethically sound for the hospital to allow an inexperienced and unlicensed student to "learn" at her expense, especially since she had suffered for more than 40 hours because of a prior surgical injury? How does a teaching hospital balance the rights of and responsibilities to its patients with providing education and training for new clinicians?

7. Since at least 2013, wide discussion has occurred in the healthcare community, as well as the media, about preventable medical errors being the third leading cause of death in the United States after heart disease and cancer. Everyone has a story about medical errors. What have you personally experienced? What stories have you have heard from instructors, colleagues, coworkers, and fellow students? Can you identify the cultural and procedural practices that enable errors to continue to happen? How does the author's story influence your opinions about medical errors?

Nursing Advocacy

"The nurse's primary commitment is to the patient, whether an individual, family, group, community, or population" (American Nurses Association, 2015, p. 5).

1. Other than her sisters and friend, did the author have anyone to advocate for her in the hospital? In what ways could the author's nurses have advocated for her after she began to experience deepening, unremitting pain after the initial surgery? Other than documenting the pain and treating it with the prescribed medication, could the nurses have done

anything else to prevent her from suffering for more than 40 hours before she was rushed back to surgery to repair her perforated bowel? What if nurses had inquired about better medicating her pain? What if they had questioned whether she might have a perforated bowel? Could their questions have made a difference in her outcome?

2. When a patient experiences questionable or poor care from anyone in the hospital, do most nurses know how to use the chain of authority to advocate for the patient? What if senior administrators do not appreciate nurses who identify systemic problems that cause or contribute to patient injuries, poor care, or worse? How can nurses be expected to tell the truth if doing so jeopardizes their jobs? What steps can nurses take to begin to change an environment of silence and fear to one of openness and accountability?

3. Explore some whistle-blower situations where nurses bravely fought for their patients' safety. (Begin with the Texas nurse whistle-blowers from this *New York Times* article if you don't know of others: http://www.nytimes.com/2010/02/12/us/12nurses.html?_r=0.) If you were in a situation where physicians, surgeons, or nurses were endangering patients, what would it take for you to blow the whistle?

4. As a nurse, nursing student, or other healthcare student or provider working in a teaching hospital, have you witnessed or heard stories that involve inexperienced or seasoned doctors or nurses who:

- Demonstrate poor or inadequate patient care?
- Work without adequate leadership and guidance?
- Appear unable or unwilling to ask for assistance from or listen to others?
- Perform in a hurried, unsafe, or incompetent manner?
- Render incomplete, inappropriate, or dangerous patient care?

- Communicate poorly, or not at all, with patients, family members, or other staff?

- Fail to demonstrate caring and compassionate care to patients or others?

The author has established an email address to collect preventable medical-error stories. Please consider sharing your story at thepatientinroom2@gmail.com.

Disclosure

1. After the author awoke from her coma and began to piece together her story, she expected the hospital to reveal why she ended up in a coma on a ventilator after five surgeries. Other than a few details from her surgeon before her discharge, she learned nothing from the hospital until 2 years later. Imagine how the author felt. More than 3 weeks of her life were completely blank. How can an institution with a deeply ingrained fear of malpractice balance the patient's right to know when errors are made with the needs of the institution to protect itself and continue to train new healthcare providers in the future? How does a teaching hospital reconcile the conflict between training new doctors and other healthcare providers with providing the best care for patients? Could transparency be part of the answer?

2. The author discusses why people choose not to sue for malpractice, even when they are fully informed of the actions that caused their suffering. Do you work in a facility that owns responsibility for its errors, or does your workplace conceal or deny errors? What are some ways that individuals can begin to change the culture of silence?

Accountability

1. The author lost a month of her life and suffered significant injuries at the hands of her surgeons and other care providers. She faced further reconstructive surgery and years of recovery. Factoring out financial recompense, what fundamental aspects of accountability did hospital administrators and surgeons owe her that they did not deliver? Imagine how your workplace would have handled a similar case. Consider and discuss how your hospital or healthcare facility could have held itself accountable in a similar situation.

2. After a month in the hospital, the author was released as if she had experienced a "normal" hospitalization. She received standard discharge information for home care, but no information about how her body might have been affected because of the physical and psychological insults she had experienced (Chapters 11 and 12). Her taste had altered, her mouth would not close during sleep, and she lost her hair, among other experiences. Did she experience substandard discharge care? Is a lack of discharge information relating to a specific patient's condition common among hospitals? Consider how your hospital handles the discharge of patients who have been very sick and/or traumatized by their care. Are they given adequate, personalized discharge information as they leave the hospital? How would you write up discharge instructions for the author?

3. Describe and discuss hospital policies that enhance transparency while lowering risks. Have any institutions successfully transformed their mission statements to improve patient safety and be more accountable to patients, while also reducing their financial risks?

Suffering

1. The author emphasizes how important it is for healthcare providers, especially nurses and doctors, to understand and address patient suffering. How do you define suffering? How do you recognize and address it in your clinical practice? Is failing to see or ameliorate a patient's suffering an ethical concern? How can a person provide care and comfort to ameliorate nonphysical suffering?

2. Suffering is not just about pain or the body; it is often existential, beyond language, invisible to others. How does the author describe the relationship between *personhood* and *suffering?* How does she suggest someone can learn to become aware of patient suffering? How is the personhood of a nurse or doctor connected to the personhood of a patient?

3. How does suffering connect us to one another? How does the author's suffering affect how she relates to her mother (Chapter 17)?

4. Define *powerlessness* in the author's situation and how it related to her suffering. Do you ever consider a patient's sense of powerlessness or hopelessness?

5. Describe the author's emotional suffering as she writes about dying (Chapters 1 and 16). What coping skills did she use?

Ego

1. Ego can be dangerous in healthcare. In the author's story, did arrogance and ego play a part in her initial injury? In the injuries that followed her first surgery? In the way hospital administrators treated her as she sought to understand what had happened to her? Many assert that physician training instills arrogance, sometimes disguised as confidence, which is commonly considered essential for accepting responsibil-

ity for patients' lives. The author discusses this as *paternalism*, which may occur, for example, when a doctor presumes to unilaterally know what is best for a patient, or when a doctor is aware of what a patient wants and disregards the patient's wishes. Have you experienced paternalism in the workplace or as a patient? Discuss how the deep-seated nature of paternalism can play a role in silencing preventable errors.

2. During the month the author was in the hospital, she experienced exceptional care as well as deeply damaging care that caused her injuries. Discuss some of the author's experiences with nurses driven by ego. Consider how the egos of various colleagues and coworkers come into play. What are the potential outcomes of unchecked egos in healthcare?

EXCEPTIONAL CARE

1. The author was traumatized by the poor quality of care she received after being admitted to the hospital. How did her traumatic experience extend to her family? What are the special care needs of patients' families, especially in regard to comatose, noncommunicative, or dying patients? Describe the concept of "family as patient" and explore the responsibilities of healthcare providers for families.

2. The author's sister later mentioned that she did not realize medicine was "all math." What did she mean by this statement? How did the "numbers game" play out in the delayed diagnosis of the author's surgical injury and in the general care she received before her emergency surgery more than 40 hours later?

3. The author's treatment consisted of multiple catheters and invasive medical devices, including central IVs, a Foley catheter, a wound vac, and a ventilator. How might each of these items contribute to a patient's risk of infection?

4. Consider the author's story *after* she was brought out of her coma and removed from the ventilator. For a while, she was awake and aware but psychotic and unable to communicate until tubes were removed from her throat. How can a nurse address a patient's sense of isolation and loneliness, especially if the patient is unable to comprehend the circumstances or does not know or remember what has happened?

5. Does a nurse's duty of care change depending on whether patients are able to understand their situation, communicate their thoughts and feelings, or remember recent events—or whether the patient is expected to recover? In what ways?

6. What are the causes, symptoms, and treatment for ICU psychosis? How common is ICU psychosis, and can it be prevented?

7. Often, patients have no memory of psychotic episodes. The author remembered much of what happened after she came off the ventilator. Knowing that, have you changed your view of how nurses need to care for critically ill and ICU patients? In what way?

8. The author never slept while in the hospital after awakening from her coma. What physical and mental factors, as well as external factors, sometimes keep patients awake in a hospital? What can hospitals do to support patients' sleep and rest? How can nurses help patients who do not sleep feel more comfortable and experience less distress?

9. Why do some patients who may know or suspect that medical errors affected their care fail to pursue answers? Consider the author, who was informed and tenacious. What about patients who are neither informed nor tenacious enough to advocate for themselves? How do they recover their story or obtain some form of justice?

10. Discuss the author's letter (Chapter 15) about her future wishes regarding surgery. Do you think it made a difference in the care she received? If so, how?

11. Consider the author's telephone interaction with the radiologist (Chapter 16) while awaiting news about potential new cancer suspicions. How did the radiologist connect with the author in a very simple way over the phone, and how did it make the author feel?

12. Think back to the story of when the author advocated for her patient while she was a nursing student (Chapter 18). How would you feel about speaking up in such a situation? Think about how you can gain the skills and confidence to become a better patient advocate. What do you need from your instructors, managers, or employer to improve your patient advocacy skills?

13. The author faced expensive dental procedures later on, due to the damage from her stay in the SICU. Could her dental problems have been prevented? Consider and discuss ways care providers can support a patient's dental hygiene to potentially prevent future reconstruction.

ETHICAL EXPLORATIONS

1. The following ethical principles are defined in the glossary: *autonomy, beneficence, fidelity, justice, nonmaleficence, and veracity.* How can healthcare providers ensure that ethical consideration is part of each patient interaction? In Chapter 18, the author explains how ignorance of how to identify and address ethical concepts in clinical practice often contributes to moral distress among nurses and other clinicians. Consider examples you have heard about, or experienced personally, when patient care was enhanced or compromised by the presence or absence of sound ethical decision-making.

2. Review the definitions of the ethical principles of *beneficence, fidelity, nonmaleficence,* and *veracity.* Which are most important to consider when caring for someone who is unconscious or who cannot communicate? Why?

3. How can ethical principles help guide nursing care for effective pain management? Give examples of specific ethical principles and situations where the pain was, or was not, effectively managed.

4. How does a nurse relate to an unconscious patient's humanity when the nurse has not met the patient before and knows nothing about the patient except the current physical picture?

5. While still in the hospital because of the medical errors (Chapter 9), the author discusses telling her surgeon that she did not want additional treatments in case she had a heart attack or stroke before she went home. Do you think she had the right to make this request? What do you think of his response that she was likely suffering depression because of her trauma? Did the surgeon have a responsibility to seriously consider her request?

6. Can a patient experience *autonomy* in an ICU? How can patients practice self-determination when they do not know what is needed to recover and get well? What part do advance directives play in a patient's healthcare decision-making process?

7. Without the patient's participation, what burden is placed on nurses, doctors, family, and others who must make care decisions?

8. Consider the practice of hospitals allowing inexperienced and potentially unskilled surgical fellows to operate (practice) on patients. One side argues that medical practitioners have to learn somehow. Another side argues that every patient has a right to the highest-quality care available. Explore how teaching hospitals can effectively instruct and train physicians and

other medical-care providers while ensuring the highest possible care to patients. When a conflict exists between doing what is best to treat and care for a patient and what is best for the hospital in training new doctors, which ethical principles are at stake? Is it ever ethically acceptable to train a doctor if the patient's safety and care will be compromised?

9. Consider which ethical principles are relevant in conflicts between healthcare costs and patient well-being.

10. Prior to her repair surgery 14 months after her monthlong hospitalization, the author encountered conflict (Chapter 15) with an anesthesiologist in a pre-op appointment. Which ethical principles did the doctor violate? Which ethical principles did the author rely on to handle the situation?

11. What is Abraham Maslow's hierarchy of needs? Where did the author's experiences fit into the hierarchy of needs when she was in the hospital? When she first came home? When she went back to work? When she had another major surgery the following year?

12. Nursing theorist Jean Watson talks about the science and art of nursing, in which the nurse brings loving kindness, authentic presence, and equanimity to the nurse-patient relationship (*see* https://www.watsoncaringscience.org/). What does Watson mean by "authentic presence"? By "equanimity" in the nurse-patient relationship? Discuss the ethical concepts related to the presence or absence of this type of caring connection. How does your nursing practice demonstrate caring for your patient? For yourself? For your colleagues?

HEALTHCARE CONSUMER'S GUIDE

1. Through trying to learn what happened to her, the author discovered that the third leading cause of death in the United States is preventable hospital medical errors and adverse events. Because this finding is based on incomplete statistics, it does not truly represent how pervasive medical errors are in our hospitals. In a recent analysis, Makary and Daniel (2016) explained that, because medical errors are not a choice for inclusion on death certificates, it is not possible to know the full extent of harm caused by medical errors. Consider stories you have heard about someone who experienced trauma or even died from poor care, medication errors, hospital-acquired infections, falls, blood clots, bed sores, pneumonia, and surgical complications, to name a few. Were they in a hospital? An outpatient office? A clinic setting? Were they having major surgery, diagnostic testing, or elective procedures?

2. Many healthcare consumers go to their medical providers, anxiously hoping to have their problem resolved as quickly as possible—not wishing to go through the discomfort of asking challenging and probing questions, especially in a fast-paced medical office or clinic. People often do not know which questions to ask, and doctors and nurses may be too busy to spend enough time to give patients more than the required information. Additionally, too few people consider getting a second opinion because they lack the time or the patience to deal with their health insurance coverage, or because they just want to resolve the situation and move on with their lives. What are the dangers of a rushed and passive approach to consuming healthcare? If you experience your healthcare this way, how does it make you feel? Would you consider changing your primary care provider to have a more open and supportive experience when you need help?

3. Having read the author's experience of preventable medical errors, consider what you might do differently if you need to

schedule surgery. Do you have advance directives (living will and healthcare power of attorney)? Have you told a friend or family member what you want if things go wrong? In the event you are unconscious and unable to act on your behalf, do you trust that your doctor and the hospital will honor your living will and healthcare power of attorney? Will your loved ones protect your wishes if you have made them known? Although the format of advance directives may vary from state to state, federal law requires that these documents be provided to consumers at no cost. No attorney is needed. After you complete the documents, all you need to do is notarize them and keep the originals in a place you can easily locate. Give copies to healthcare providers when appropriate.

4. Describe the difference between a living will and healthcare power of attorney. Do you consider yourself too young to execute these documents? Many people who survive traumatic accidents and end up in a persistent vegetative state had not considered creating advance directives because they thought they were too young to die.

5. If you create an advance directive, be sure to also inform your family and loved ones about your wishes. Because most people are uncomfortable talking about death and dying, they are unlikely to have family discussions about these issues until there is an emergency situation. Yet, most people will say they never want medical technology—such as ventilators or feeding tubes—to keep them alive, especially if they are brain-dead. If you do not have advance directives, would members of your family disagree about what you would want? Having your wishes documented can help ensure you will get the care you want, while sparing loved ones of having to make difficult decisions they may be unable or unwilling to make. Generally, patients are left on machines in the absence of clear directives to take them off.

6. If you could have only one advance directive—a living will or a healthcare power of attorney—which would give you the most protection? Do you know whom you would ask to speak for you? Do you feel comfortable discussing these sensitive health issues with that person? Would you consider organizing a family meeting to talk about quality of life and the care each member would choose to have at the end of life?

7. What is the relationship between patient autonomy and advance directives? When is an advance directive activated?

8. Would you trust your hospital to deliver safe, high-quality care if you got sick? If you could choose among several hospitals near you, would you trust the hospital that had the highest safety record? You can research this at http://www.hospitalsafetyscore.org/. Which hospital would you go to in your area and why? Is your decision based on ratings? Personal experience? Family or community history?

REFERENCES

Agency for Healthcare Research and Quality. (2014). *Never events*. Retrieved from https://psnet.ahrq.gov/primers/primer/3/never-events

American Cancer Society. (2016). Cancer type: Uterine corpus. Retrieved from https://cancerstatisticscenter.cancer.org/?_ga=1.260922509.183064187.145988720 2#/cancer-site/Uterine%20corpus

American Nurses Association. (2011). Justice is served: Texas physician pleads guilty. Retrieved from http://nursingworld.org/FunctionalMenuCategories/ MediaResources/PressReleases/2011-PR/Justice-is-Served-Texas-Physician-Pleads-Guilty.pdf

American Nurses Association. (2015). *Code of ethics for nurses with interpretive statements*. Silver Spring, MD: Author.

Andel, C., Davidow, S. L., Hollander, M., & Moreno, D. A. (2012). The economics of health care quality and medical errors. *Journal of Health Care Finance, 39*(1), 39-50.

Bal, B. S. (2009). An introduction to medical malpractice in the United States. *Clinical Orthopaedics and Related Research, 467*(2), 339-347.

Boothman, R. C., & Hoyler, M. M. (2013). The University of Michigan's easy disclosure and offer program. *Bulletin of the American College of Surgeons, 98*(3), 21-25.

Boothman, R. C., Imhoff, S. J., & Campbell, D. A. (2012). Nurturing a culture of patient safety and achieving lower malpractice risk through disclosure: Lessons learned and future directions. *Frontiers of Health Services Management, 28*(3), 13-28.

Cassell, E. J. (1991). *The nature of suffering and the goals of medicine*. New York, NY: Oxford University Press.

Cassell, E. J. (1999). Diagnosing suffering: A perspective. *Annals of Internal Medicine, 131*(7), 531-534.

Cassell, E. J. (2010). The person in medicine. *International Journal of Integrative Care, 10*(Suppl.), e019. Retrieved from http://www.ncbi.nlm.nih.gov/pmc/articles/ PMC2834910

Cavallazzi, R., Saad, M., & Marik, P. E. (2012). Delirium in the ICU: An overview. *Annals of Intensive Care, 2*(49). Retrieved from http://annalsofintensivecare.springeropen.com/articles/10.1186/2110-5820-2-49

Centers for Disease Control and Prevention. (2016). National and state healthcare acquired infections progress report. Retrieved from http://www.cdc.gov/HAI/ pdfs/progress-report/hai-progress-report.pdf

Centers for Disease Control and Prevention. (2016, March 2). Healthcare-associated infections. Retrieved from http://www.cdc.gov/hai/surveillance/index.html

Department of Health and Human Services. (2010). Adverse events in hospitals: National incidence among Medicare beneficiaries. Retrieved from http://sma.org/michaelcgosney/files/2010/11/HHS_IG_AdverseHospEvents.pdf

Der Bedrosian, J. (2015, Summer). Nursing is hard. Unaddressed ethical issues make it even harder. *Johns Hopkins Magazine*. Retrieved from http://hub.jhu.edu/magazine/2015/summer/nursing-ethics-and-burnout

Edwin, A. K. (2009). Non-disclosure of medical errors an egregious violation of ethical principles. *Ghana Medical Journal, 43*(1), 34-39.

Epstein, E. G., & Delgado, S. (2010). Understanding and addressing moral distress. *OJIN: The Online Journal of Issues in Nursing, 15*(3). doi:10.3912/OJIN.Vol15No-03Man01

Feng, P., Huang, L., & Wang, H. (2013). Taste bud homeostasis in health, disease, and aging. *Chemical Senses, 39*(1), 3-16. doi:10.1093/chemse/bjt059

Gawande, A. (2007, December 10). The checklist. *The New Yorker.* Retrieved from http://www.newyorker.com/magazine/2007/12/10/the-checklist

Hoban, Rose. (2005, August 12). Duke patients angry at hydraulic fluid mix-up. *National Public Radio.* Retrieved from http://www.npr.org/templates/story/story.php?storyId=4797392

James, J. T. (2013). A new, evidence-based estimate of patient harms associated with hospital care. *Journal of Patient Safety, 9*(3), 122-128. doi:10.1097/PTS.0b013e3182948a69

Jena, A. B., Seabury, S., Lakdawalla, D., & Chandra, A. (2011). Malpractice risk according to physician specialty. *New England Journal of Medicine, 365*, 629-636.

Kao, K.-C., Hu, H.-C., Hsieh, M.-J., Tsai, Y.-H., & Huang, C.-C. (2015). Comparison of community-acquired, hospital-acquired, and intensive care unit-acquired acute respiratory distress syndrome: A prospective observational cohort study. *Critical Care, 19*, 384. doi:10.1186/s13054-015-1096-1

Kirchheimer, S. (2013, June). Avoid the hospital in July: Why? New doctors and nurses report to work for the first time. AARP. Retrieved from http://www.aarp.org/health/doctors-hospitals/info-06-2010/why_you_should_avoid_the_hospital_in_july.html

Kohn, L. T., Corrigan, J. M., & Donaldson, M. S. (2000). *To err is human: Building a safer health system.* Washington, DC: National Academies Press.

Landrigan, C. P., Parry, G. J., Bones, C. B., Hackbarth, A. D., Goldmann, D. A., & Sharek, P. J. (2010). Temporal trends in rates of patient harm resulting from medical care. *New England Journal of Medicine, 363*, 2124-2134. doi:10.1056/NEJMsa1004404

Magill, S. S., Edwards, J. R., Bamberg, W., Beldavs, Z. G., Dumyati, G., Kainer, M. A.
... Fridkin, S. K. (2014). Multistate point-prevalence survey of health care–associated infections. *New England Journal of Medicine, 370*(13), 1198-1208. doi:10.1056/NEJMoa1306801

Makary, M. A., & Daniel, M. (2016). Medical error—the third leading cause of death in the US. *BMJ.* doi:10.1136/bmj.i2139

Mattar, S. G., Alseidi, A. A., Jones, D. B., Jeyarajah, D. R., Swanstrom, L. L., Aye, R. W. . . . Minter, R. M. (2013). General surgery residency inadequately prepares trainees for fellowship: Results of a survey of fellowship program directors. *Annals of Surgery, 258*(3), 440-449. doi:10.1097/SLA.0b013e3182a191ca

Mazor, K. M., Reed, G. W., Yood, R. A., Fischer, M. A., Baril, J., & Gurwitz, J. H. (2006). Disclosure of medical errors: What factors influence how patients respond? *Journal of General Internal Medicine, (21)*7, 704-710.

O'Connor, A. (2011, September 1). Getting doctors to wash their hands. *The New York Times.* Retrieved from http://well.blogs.nytimes.com/2011/09/01/getting-doctors-to-wash-their-hands/?_r=0

Okuyama, A., Wagner, C., & Bijnen, B. (2014). Speaking up for patient safety by hospital-based health care professionals: A literature review. *BMC Health Services Research, 14*(61). doi:10.1186/1472-6963-14-61

Peck, M. S. (1978). *The road less traveled.* New York, NY: Simon & Schuster.

Ranum, D., Ma, H., Shapiro, F. E., Chang, B., & Urman, R. D. (2014). Analysis of patient injury based on anesthesiology closed claims data from a major malpractice insurer. *Journal of Healthcare Risk Management, 34*(2), 31-42. doi:10.1002/jhrm.21156

Robbins, A. (2015, May 28). We need more nurses. *The New York Times.* Retrieved from http://www.nytimes.com/2015/05/28/opinion/we-need-more-nurses.html?_r=0

Robert Wood Johnson Foundation. (2012, August 28). Better environments for nurses mean fewer medication errors. Retrieved from http://www.rwjf.org/en/library/articles-and-news/2012/08/better-environments-for-nurses-mean-fewer-medication-errors.html

Schniederjan, S., & Donovan, G. K. (2005). Ethics versus education: Pelvic exams on anesthetized women. *OSMA: Journal of the Oklahoma State Medical Association, 98*(8), 386-388.

State Center for Health Statistics. (2010, April). *Cancer incidence in North Carolina 2007.* Retrieved from http://www.schs.state.nc.us/schs/ccr/incidence07/incidence2007.pdf

U. S. Senate. (2014, July 17). *More than 1,000 preventable deaths a day is too many: The need to improve patient safety* (Senate Hearing 113-787). Washington, DC: Government Printing Office. Retrieved from https://www.gpo.gov/fdsys/pkg/CHRG-113shrg88894/html/CHRG-113shrg88894.htm

Whitehead, P. B., Herbertson, R. K., Hamric, A. B., Epstein, E. G., & Fisher, J. M. (2015). Moral distress among healthcare professionals: Report of an institution-wide survey. *Journal of Nursing Scholarship, 47*(2), 117-125. doi:10.1111/jnu.12115

Young, J. Q., Ranji, S. R., Wachter, R. M., Lee, C. M., Niehaus, B., & Auerbach, A. D. (2011). "July effect": Impact of the academic year-end changeover on patient outcomes: A systematic review. *Annals of Internal Medicine, 155*(5), 309-315. doi:10.7326/0003-4819-155-5-201109060-00354

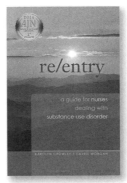
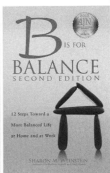
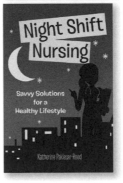
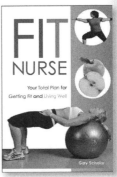

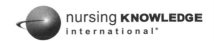

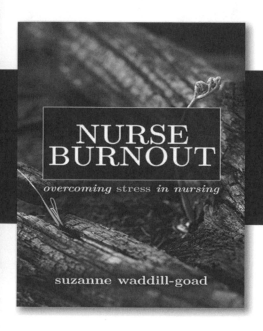

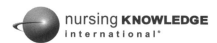

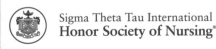
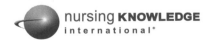

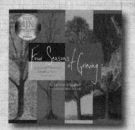
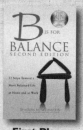
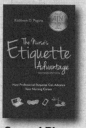
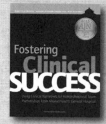
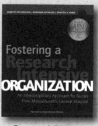
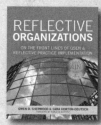
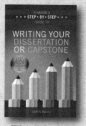

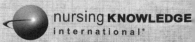